Rethinking Health Care Policy

The New Politics of State Regulation

American Governance and Public Policy

A SERIES EDITED BY

Barry Rabe and John Tierney

This series examines a broad range of public policy issues and their relationship to all levels of government in the United States. The editors welcome serious scholarly studies and seek to publish books that appeal to both academic and professional audiences. The series showcases studies that illuminate the successes, as well as the problems, of policy formulation and implementation.

Rethinking Health Care Policy

The New Politics of State Regulation

Robert B. Hackey

GEORGETOWN UNIVERSITY PRESS / WASHINGTON, D.C.

Georgetown University Press, Washington, D.C. 20007
© 1998 by Georgetown University Press. All rights reserved.

10 9 8 7 6 5 4 3 2 1   1998

Library of Congress Cataloging-in-Publication Data

Hackey, Robert B.
   Rethinking health care policy : the new politics of state
regulation / Robert B. Hackey.
      p.   cm. — (American governance and public policy)
   Includes bibliographical references and index.
   1. Hospital care—Cost control—Government policy—United States—
States.   I. Title.   II. Series.
RA981.A2H27   1998
362.1′1′0973—dc21   97-37198
ISBN 0-87840-668-9 (cloth).
ISBN 0-87840-669-7 (paper)

For Tacy and Meagan, with love.

Contents

Acknowledgments

I have lived with the research presented in this book for more than five years. The arguments raised herein were first presented, in skeletal form, as a graduate paper in Jim Morone's health policy seminar at Brown University. Jim sparked my interest in health care politics and policy when I was a graduate student; as my thesis advisor, he encouraged me to "look at the big picture" without losing sight of the details. The thoughtful contributions of many colleagues are much appreciated. I am particularly indebted to Chris Bosso and Michael Dukakis of Northeastern University and Larry Weil of Rhode Island College for their willingness to provide helpful comments and feedback on previous drafts of the manuscript.

My research introduced me to a wide range of state policymakers in the Northeastern states. As a graduate student, and later as a health planner in Rhode Island, I developed an enormous respect for the professionalism and dedication of those who work in state regulatory agencies. Without their generous contribution of time, insights, and data, this book would not have been possible. In particular, I am indebted to many colleagues who read and commented on earlier versions of the manuscript. At the Rhode Island Department of Health, Bill Waters and Don Williams offered encouragement and incisive critiques of my work on state certificate-of-need and health planning programs. Michael McMullan and Gloria Smiddy of the U.S. Health Care Financing Administration provided me with reams of data on state Medicaid program expenditures and state waiver applications.

My views on state policy-making and regulatory politics were also shaped by the comments of numerous external reviewers who critiqued earlier versions of my argument published in *Medical Care Review; The Journal of Health Politics, Policy, and Law;* and *Spectrum: The Journal of State Government.* In particular, my initial attempt to develop a regime-based model of policy choice appeared in *Medical Care Review* 49 (Fall 1992) as "Trapped Between State and Market: Regulating Hospital Reimbursement in the Northeastern States." A revised version of this argument was subsequently published in the *Journal of Health Politics, Policy, and Law* 18 (Summer 1993) as "Regulatory Regimes and State

Cost Containment Programs." My first efforts to grapple with the political dynamics of state certificate-of-need (CON) programs also appeared in the *Journal of Health Politics, Policy, and Law* 18 (Winter 1993) as "New wine in Old Bottles: Certificate of Need Enters the 1990s." Finally, an overview of Rhode Island's experience with prospective rate-setting was published in *Spectrum* 69 (Winter 1996) as "Setting Limits Through Global Budgeting: Hospital Cost Containment in Rhode Island."

I have also benefited from a remarkable group of academic colleagues and generous support from administrators at both St. Anselm College and the University of Massachusetts Dartmouth. The enthusiastic support of Rev. Peter J. Guerin, the Dean of the College at St. Anselm, enabled me to finish my thesis, pay my bills, and present the first fruits of my research to the 1991 Annual Meeting of the American Political Science Association. At UMass-Dartmouth, my conversations with Clyde Barrow about state capacity, state autonomy, and the conceptual issues in contemporary state theory helped to define the theoretical framework presented in the first two chapters. In addition, as director of the Center for Policy Analysis, Clyde generously provided release time during the 1994–95 academic year. As department chair, Jean Doyle has been a vital source of support and encouragement; her willingness to craft imaginative teaching schedules for me over the past two years hastened the completion of revisions by many months. Frank Corey, Nancy Farias, Jeff Guilbault, Brian King, and Joe Wagner spent many hours toiling in the library's microfilm room on my behalf; their efforts are much appreciated. My analysis of policy regimes also benefited from my interactions with three unusually talented graduate students at the University of Rhode Island; Peter Fuller, Dave DeSousa, and Pam Whitehouse pushed me to tie up loose ends and probed for theoretical weaknesses in my argument. Their contributions are most appreciated.

My deepest debts, however, are to the many public and private officials who agreed to be interviewed for this project. Quotations which appear in the following chapters were drawn from a series of semi-structured interviews conducted during the summer of 1990 and the spring of 1992 in Massachusetts, New Hampshire, New York, and Rhode Island. Since respondents were guaranteed anonymity to secure candid responses about topics controversial within their organizations, their names do not appear in the text. Special thanks to Steve Anderman, Barry Bodell, Jay Buechner, Jim Carney, Stephen Cleary, Michael Cook, Alain Couture, Bruce Cryan, John Daley, Mike Dexter, John Donahue, Stanley Duncan, Don Ford, Jack Grant, Paula Griswold, Brian Hendricks, Darrell Jeffers, Brian Keeler, Melinda Komiske, Thomas Lynch, Bob Menard, Richard Michel, Mark Montella, Robert Padpug,

Martha Pofit, Karen Quigley, Elliot Shaw, Al Smith, Mark Thomas, John Wardle, Bill Waters, Don Williams, and Ed Zesk. John Dickens, Ed Duschesne, William Gormley, Joyce James, Stan Lane, and John Scioli all provided essential data on the performance of CON programs in their states. Without their generous contributions of time and data, this manuscript would not have been possible.

Publishing a book for the first time is never an easy task. My conversations with numerous colleagues during the many months of writing and revising this manuscript led me to greatly appreciate the nurturing and supportive environment at Georgetown University Press. John Samples invited me to submit a manuscript to the press' new series, offered continuing support as I prepared the first draft of the manuscript, and provided a much needed voice of encouragement during the process of revision. Patricia Rayner and the production staff at the press significantly improved the flow of the manuscript and patiently endured my tendency to let deadlines slip. I will always be grateful for their efforts and guidance.

Other debts, however, are more personal. Barbara Harris diligently read every word of this manuscript several times during its transformation from a thesis to a book. Her constant reminders to consider my audience, avoid the passive voice, and tighten up my writing contributed to the readability of the chapters which follow. I am forever in her debt for her patience and the generous gift of her time. Any theoretical shortcomings or other oversights in the pages that follow, however, are my own. My heartiest thanks must go to my wife, Tacy, who has lived with me and this book, for the past five years. As she will attest, it wasn't always easy. As a small token of my appreciation for all that she's done, this book is dedicated to her, and to our daughter Meagan, with many, many thanks for their patience.

1

States and the Health Care Crisis

"Our health care system is broken. If we go on without change, the consequences will be devastating for millions of Americans and disastrous for the nation in human and economic terms." Hillary Rodham Clinton, 1994.

"Today millions of Americans cannot afford the health care they need and are forced to choose between the sickbed and the poorhouse." Sen. Henry M. Jackson (D-WA), 1976.

"The insecurity caused by the health crisis in America gnaws at the American family and at the deepest roots of our society." Leonard Woodcock, chairman of the Committee for National Health Insurance, 1970.

Politicians, pundits, and health care providers have warned for more than three decades that the U.S. health care system was "poised on the verge of a . . . meltdown" (Lundberg 1992). In the 1960s and early 1970s, the principal concern among reformers was ensuring access to care for uninsured and underserved populations. By the 1980s, the focus of health care reform efforts had shifted to cost containment, as health care inflation reached "unsustainable" levels. The rising cost of medical care was reflected in exploding Medicaid budgets, higher taxes, cutbacks in domestic spending in other policy domains, and growing concerns about the economic competitiveness of American industry. The 1990s brought a new set of concerns. As managed care organizations (MCOs) applied new pressures on hospitals to control costs, consumers, physicians, and public officials clamored for new regulations to ensure that the cost-containment strategies employed by providers and third-party insurers would not undermine the quality of patient care. Continuing concerns about the state of the nation's health care system generated many promises from presidents and congressional leaders to enact comprehensive reform at the federal level, but produced few concrete results. In the absence of comprehensive national health care reform, state governments emerged as the principal source of policy innovation in health care policy-making.

Despite common agreement over the need for reform, states have followed markedly different routes to control costs, increase access to health care, and monitor the quality of health care services. A number of states experimented with comprehensive reform programs in the late 1980s and early 1990s, but persistent implementation and financing problems stalled most state efforts to achieve universal coverage or restructure how hospitals and providers were paid. In particular, several sweeping reform initiatives that proposed to implement statewide global budgets or expenditure caps for hospital and health care services (e.g., in Minnesota, New York, Vermont, and Washington) were scaled back or abandoned soon after they were enacted. State efforts to guarantee access to health care through employer mandated health insurance or uncompensated care pools (e.g., Massachusetts, New Jersey, and New York) also ran afoul of the provisions of the Employee Retirement and Income Security Act of 1974 (ERISA).[1] In spite of these setbacks, however, state interest in health care reform remains high, and cost containment commands attention from a growing cadre of health policy specialists in state legislatures, health departments, and private sector interest groups.

This book develops an analytical model to compare differences in the policy choices, implementation, and outcomes of state initiatives to control hospital costs. Interactions between public officials and health care providers reflect the larger relationship between state government and the private sector, for the development and implementation of health care regulatory policies occur in the context of a state's prevailing political culture and institutions. The design of political institutions, the policy preferences and economic interests of public and private decision makers, and the resources available to public officials all influence the nature, timing, and effectiveness of state regulatory efforts. Since both political culture and the autonomy and capacity of political institutions vary from state to state, different policy environments will produce different approaches to cost containment and different policy outcomes. In this context, the autonomy, capacity, and legitimacy of state political institutions is as important as the adoption of a particular reimbursement methodology or capital expenditure threshold in determining the success or failure of state regulatory programs (Hackey 1992).

With few exceptions (Brown 1993; Morone and Dunham 1983; Morone 1990; Thompson 1981), political explanations of the evolution and performance of state health care regulation have been conspicuously absent. As a result, no framework presently exists to account for "who gets what, when, and how" in state health care policy. Given the breadth and scope of current state reform proposals, the absence of an accurate portrait of the administrative and regulatory capacities of state governments is a critical shortcoming of the current literature on health care policy-making. Continued enthusiasm for state-level health care reform raises important questions about this administrative and regulatory capacity of state governments. Is it realistic to expect states to undertake new tasks at a time when they have been burdened by budget crises and a wide range of unfunded federal mandates? Critics contend that most states lack both the financial and administrative resources needed to improve access to health care for the uninsured or to bring costs under control (see Thompson 1986; Sapolsky 1986; Stone 1992). In particular, state efforts to expand access to health care to underserved and uninsured populations have often been handicapped by a lack of resources. After auspicious beginnings earlier in the decade, bold reform plans in Minnesota, Vermont, and Washington were either scuttled entirely or significantly reduced in scope after 1994.

A close examination of state efforts to control health care costs over the past two decades provides a natural experiment to explore the formulation and implementation of a wide range of policy instruments. As such, state health care policy can improve our understanding of several conceptual issues in the study of state politics. In particular, the diversity of responses to rising health care costs offers an opportunity to explore cross-sectional variation in policy adoption and implementation issues as well as rapid changes in policy over time (e.g., deregulation in rate-setting states). The diversity of state responses to the emerging crisis in health care, however, presents a policy paradox. Why did some states opt for regulatory controls, while others enlisted the support of private interests to control costs, and still others ceded control over health care policy-making to providers?

To answer these questions, the following chapters present a comparative case study of health care policy-making in four Northeastern states—Massachusetts, New Hampshire, New York, and Rhode Island—which followed different paths to controlling health care costs over the past two decades. A comparative case study design provides an opportunity to capture the process of coalition formation and bargaining within policy subsystems using multiple data sources (Stonecash 1996; Yin 1989). Although all of the states share a number of important characteristics (e.g., region, approval for Medicaid 1115 waivers), each has had markedly different experiences with health care regulation over the past two decades. In New Hampshire and Rhode Island, health care policy-making emerged through a collaborative and relatively nonconflictual process; once established, the system of health care financing in each state proved to be remarkably stable. In contrast, Massachusetts and New York were early leaders in hospital rate setting and certificate-of-need regulation, but both opted to deregulate their hospital payment systems in the 1990s. Furthermore, while health care policy-making has been a low-visibility issue in New Hampshire and Rhode Island, health care regulation has been a highly contentious topic in Massachusetts and New York over the past two decades.

James Q. Wilson's (1986) observation that several basic questions about the politics of regulation remain either unanswered or unexplored is still true today. In particular, few studies have examined when and why governments decide to intervene in the operation of free markets (Wilson 1986, 357). This question is particularly relevant for the study of health care regulation, for states have pursued very different paths to control the common problem of rising health care costs over the past two decades. A number of basic questions concerning the relative merits of regulation versus competition as a cost-control strategy remain unanswered. For example, what factors affect a state's choice of cost-containment strategies? Why have some states embraced strict regulatory controls, while others have been content to follow a hands-off, market-oriented strategy? Why are hospital reimbursement issues hotly contested in some states but not in others? In other words, how can we account for the different political dynamics among states which have adopted similar regulatory strategies? Finally, under what circumstances are state governments able to effectively control hospital costs? Each of the following chapters returns to these questions in an effort to provide an understanding of the political dynamics beneath the surface of state health care policy-making.

STATE APPROACHES TO CONTROLLING HEALTH CARE COSTS

States embraced a variety of policy instruments in their quest to control the rising cost of health care. During the 1970s and early 1980s, states turned to two related, yet distinct, regulatory strategies to control spiraling hospital costs. Hospitals received the lion's share of attention from policymakers over the past two decades because payments to hospitals are by far the largest single category of health care expenditures. The first approach, hospital rate regulation, sought to control costs by limiting the amount providers could charge patients and third party insurers; the second, health planning and certificate-of-need regulation, attempted to limit the construction of new health care facilities and the diffusion of new technologies to "appropriate" levels consistent with the goals outlined in a statewide health plan. While a number of states achieved considerable success in controlling health care costs through regulation (Hadley and Swartz 1989; Robinson and Luft 1988; Thorpe 1993), such programs often encountered strong opposition from health care providers.

Rate-Setting

Hospital rate regulation first gained popularity as a cost-control strategy in the 1970s, when federal and state governments extended their authority over both facilities expansion and provider reimbursement under the aegis of health planning and rate-setting programs. Hospitals have received the lion's share of attention from policymakers interested in controlling health care costs. Payments to hospitals are by far the largest single category of health care expenditures and accounted for nearly one half (44%) of all personal health care spending in 1991 (Letsch 1993). Hospital payments also present a particularly inviting target for government regulation because they have exceeded the rate of overall medical inflation over the past two decades (HCFA 1988). Although early studies of the effects of state hospital regulation yielded mixed evidence (Sloan 1981; Eby and Cohodes 1985), more recent studies have demonstrated that rate-setting programs were more effective than competitive strategies in controlling hospital costs (Robinson and Luft 1988; Hadley and Swartz 1989).

Knowledge of the regulatory process under such programs, however, remains cursory. To date, most studies of state hospital rate-setting programs have neglected political explanations and have focused on variables such as the unit of revenue subject to regulation, the basis of payment, or the system's scope as the principal determinants of regulatory success or failure (Biles et al. 1980; Hellinger 1985; Hadley and Swartz 1989; Sloan 1983; Sloan 1981). By the early 1990s, the issue seemed to be a moot point, as many observers argued that the heyday of regulation had passed (McDonough 1995). Several states which had pursued a rate-setting approach to hospital cost containment deregulated their payment systems in the 1980s; several other states followed suit in the early 1990s. Rumors of the demise of regulation, however, may be premature. Several states considered legislation which would establish statewide global budgets for health services (e.g., New York), single-payer financing systems (e.g., Vermont), or regulated all-payer rate-setting systems (e.g., Montana, Vermont) during 1994 and 1995. Instead of fading away, the nature of state regulation of health care providers and insurers is changing in the 1990s in response to underlying shifts in the organization and delivery of health care services.

Rate-setting programs proliferated in the 1970s and early 1980s; by 1985, fourteen states used diagnosis-related groups to determine Medicaid payments for inpatient hospital care, while seven states had adopted all-payer rate-setting programs that established standards of reimbursement for all third-party insurers (Perkins 1985). From their inception, hospital rate-setting programs attracted both strong defenders and passionate detractors. Rate regulation was hailed by proponents as a solution to rampant health care inflation that offered state officials the means to curb double-digit increases in Medicaid expenditures and health insurance premiums and subsidize care for the uninsured. Critics, however, contended that such programs were inefficient at best, or threatened the managerial discretion of administrators and the continued fiscal health of hospitals in regulated areas.

Empirical studies of hospital regulation over the past two decades further muddied the debate over the relative merits of rate-setting and competition as cost-control strategies, for state regulatory programs varied widely in both scope and effectiveness. After more than a decade of experimentation with various forms of prospective reimbursement, programs in New York, Maryland, and Massachusetts generated impressive cost savings, while others did not (Eby and Cohodes 1985; Thorpe 1993). After decades of trying to avoid government intervention and maintain autonomy, the hospital industry in many states now resembles a quasi-public utility whose profits and operating conditions are largely determined by the actions of state regulatory agencies.

Certificate-of-Need Regulation

In the eyes of their critics, certificate-of-need (CON) programs have failed to control costs, stifled competition (Burda 1991), and had little impact on access to health care for either the poor or geographically underserved regions (Sloan 1988). Indeed, Randall Bovbjerg (1988, 206) argues that "the evidence that CON in practice has accomplished any useful social objectives is very weak." Current perceptions of CON's failure as a cost-control strategy, however, are based largely on assessments of program performance during the 1970s (Salkever and Bice 1981; Sloan 1988). Although few scholars have explored the experiences of state certificate-of-need programs in the 1980s and 1990s, more recent evidence suggests that the performance of many CON programs has improved over time (Hackey 1993; Donahue et al. 1992). The expiration of the federal Health Planning and Resource Development Act (Pub. L. 93–641) in 1986 produced a wide range of responses among the states: twelve states abandoned CON altogether, others raised the threshold for CON review, and still others strengthened their programs. In addition, at least one state (New Jersey) has taken steps to recreate local planning agencies to review capital projects (Brandon 1991).

Critics of capital expenditure regulation contend that hospitals often supported CON review as a less onerous alternative to prospective rate setting programs. However, several states that pioneered CON legislation prior to the passage of federal health planning legislation in 1974 were also early leaders in hospital rate regulation (e.g., Massachusetts, New Jersey, New York, Rhode Island). Early assessments of program performance generally concluded that CON had little impact on overall hospital cost inflation, but the experiences of several states that implemented capital expenditure caps over the past decade suggest that CON's limitations as a cost-control strategy are related to "the lack of competition for a limited pool of resources" (Young 1991, 272). Under an open-ended CON review process, an unlimited number of projects could be approved if applicants could demonstrate that the proposed services were "needed." A ceiling on capital expenditures forces decision makers to prioritize programs and choose those projects that offer the greatest benefits (Young 1991; Donahue et al. 1992). Since the merits of each institution's application are judged relative to others, the implementation of a capital cap creates a zero-sum game for providers in which the approval of one project automatically reduces the funds available for others.[2] As a policy tool, however, CON programs remain unpopular with providers and are limited in their ability to change the behavior of health care providers.

Competition

Market competition, rather than government price and entry regulation, emerged as the preferred means of controlling health care costs over the past decade. Alain Enthoven, Mark Pauly, and other proponents of competition argued that government regulation had contributed to the cost spiral by inhibiting competition among health care providers. In this view, the best route to improving the efficiency of the U.S. health care system was to encourage firms and individuals to become "prudent purchasers" of health care (Dranove 1993; Enthoven and Kronick 1989a, 1989b; Pauly et al. 1991). To date, however, the impact of managed care on health care costs remains uncertain, for while competition appears to have reduced costs in some markets, in others MCOs appear to "shadow price" traditional indemnity plans in order to gain market share (Luft, Maerki, and Trauner 1986; Johnson and Aquilina 1986; Robinson 1991).

The rapid growth of managed care in the 1980s reshaped the organization and delivery of health care services throughout the United States. Managed care organizations range from traditional "group practice" health maintenance organizations (HMOs) to "open panel" independent practice associations (IPAs), preferred provider organizations (PPOs), "managed indemnity" plans, and point-of-service (POS) plans that allow patients more choice to see providers outside of a limited provider network at a higher cost. All forms of managed care, however, seek to control costs by limiting the utilization of health care services and encouraging patients to use "preferred" providers who agree to comply with the plan's practice standards and utilization controls (Weiner and de Lissovoy 1993). The growth of managed care promised states a new alternative to control costs, for hospitals and other health care providers had a strong incentive to negotiate competitive rates with MCOs. Rising HMO penetration led many state policymakers to believe that it was possible to control health care costs with little or no government involvement by fostering competition in previously stagnant health care markets. Market-oriented reforms, however, frequently required state support, for competition among health care providers before the 1980s typically centered on prestige and reputation rather than price. State efforts to foster competition among health care providers bears a strong resemblance to Ikenberry's (1988, 44) description of U.S. energy policy, for "the move toward market pricing itself required vigorous state action." States followed three distinct paths in an effort to promote competition in the health care marketplace.

The most common path was for states to seek permission from the federal government to restructure their Medicaid programs by enrolling beneficiaries in capitated MCOs. Arizona (which had been the only state in the U.S. without a Medicaid program) pioneered a new approach to cost containment by enrolling all of its Medicaid-eligible population in managed care organizations under a federal demonstration waiver from the Health Care Financing Administration (HCFA), approved in 1982 (Brecher 1984). Other states soon followed Arizona's lead; by 1996, HCFA had approved more than ninety "freedom of choice" Medicaid waivers that allowed states to enroll beneficiaries in managed care plans (Rosenbaum and Darnell 1995). At the end of 1995, more than 3.2 million Medicaid beneficiaries were enrolled in managed care plans.

With the exception of Arizona, however, most waivers granted by HCFA relied upon the limited demonstration authority granted by Section 1915 of the Social Security Act.[3] Medicaid waivers granted under Section 1915, however, were limited in scope, and did not permit states to tighten program eligibility rules, change minimum benefits, or waive federal standards for participating managed care plans. In addition, state waivers required federal approval and were limited in duration; until 1993, federal officials were reluctant to grant the more extensive Section 1115 waivers that permitted states to change federal eligibility criteria and benefit standards and modify provider payment rules (Rosenbaum and Darnell 1995). As a result, more than a decade passed after Arizona's decision to embrace Medicaid managed care before a significant number of other states turned to managed care as their principal cost-containment strategy.

Several states also sought to harness the power of market competition to transform the relationship between patients, providers, and third-party payers by increasing the purchasing power of businesses and individuals. In some states (e.g., Massachusetts), public agencies joined existing purchasing pools formed by private employers or created new public/private partnerships to purchase care (e.g., Minnesota). Elsewhere, however, alliances principally represented state and local employees (e.g., California). In Florida, Iowa, and several other states, voluntary local or regional purchasing alliances of employers and business health care coalitions sought to reshape local health care markets by becoming "prudent purchasers" of care. Considerable variation existed among the states that experimented with "managed competition," in which publicly sponsored health insurance purchasing cooperatives (HIPCs) selectively contracted with health care providers to offer a standard package of benefits. The degree of public sponsorship and regulation varied from state to state, but proponents of a pro-competitive strategy shared a common desire to shift the balance of power in health care financing from providers to "consumers" of care.

Building upon the work of Alain Enthoven and Richard Kronick, supporters of managed competition argued for insurance market reforms that would standardize benefit packages among various health insurance plans, permit open enrollment, and offer community-rated premiums to subscribers. In addition to standardizing health plans, however, more than twenty states had passed legislation to encourage the development of purchasing alliances among employers, self-insured patients, and public employees by 1996. By offering consumers a choice of health plans, each of which provided a core set of services, HIPCs encouraged the development of price competition among insurers. To attract subscribers, participating health plans had strong incentives to lower their costs by negotiating discounts with health care providers. In some states, purchasing cooperatives emerged through local, regional, or statewide business health care coalitions, with little direct involvement from state government. Elsewhere, however, states opted to create public/private purchasing alliances on a regional basis. Other states sought to implement Enthoven and Kronick's (1989a, 1989b) call for "competition under a budget" by imposing a cap on the growth of insurance premiums (e.g., Washington) or setting a statewide global budget for health care services.

In sharp contrast to reforms that sought to increase the purchasing power of employers and other consumers by creating larger purchasing pools, several states embraced a decentralized approach to stimulating competition in the health care marketplace. Despite intense opposition from health insurers, Michigan joined five other states that enacted legislation which permitted employers to offer workers "medical savings accounts" (MSAs). Under this strategy, all employees would receive a bare-bones health insurance plan to protect against the cost of catastrophic illness. Rather than relying upon competition among health care plans and providers to lower costs, however, supporters of MSAs argued that employees would have a strong incentive to limit their utilization of health care services if they paid for routine costs on an out-of-pocket basis through a designated savings account. To date, however, concerns over equity and the lack of federal tax exemptions for MSAs have limited their appeal as a policy tool.

The growing importance of state governments in formulating and implementing health care reform proposals, however, draws attention to the dearth of knowledge about state health care policy-making. More than ten years ago, Malcolm Jewell described the study of state politics as "barren" in its theoretical development (1982, 651). The same critique could be leveled against the existing literature on state health care policy, for as Sparer (1996, 192) notes, "the literature on state health governance is surprisingly thin." Investigators have typically used a single case study approach to draw conclusions about the efficacy of various policy options or the broader political environment. Since few comparative studies of state health care policy-making exist, knowledge about the politics of the regulatory process is typically drawn from individual and often idiosyncratic cases (e.g., New Jersey).[4] Depending upon which state's experience is cited, policymakers and academic observers draw vastly different conclusions about the lessons of state reform efforts. Observers are left with the difficult task of comparing research gathered on similar topics using different analytical assumptions and methods of inquiry. Although the politics of state health care regulation includes comprehensive health planning, capital expenditure regulations, hospital rate-setting programs, and global budgeting, few scholars have explored the linkage between these different—yet related—policy arenas (see Brown 1993 and Kinney 1987 for notable exceptions). At a time when Congress and many governors are clamoring for greater state autonomy over health care policy, the effect of changes in institutional structures and the process of interest group intermediation at the state level remain largely unexplored.

THE CHANGING RELATIONSHIP BETWEEN STATE GOVERNMENTS AND HEALTH CARE PROVIDERS

The health care cost explosion after 1965 fundamentally changed the relationship between state officials and health care providers. For much of the postwar period, additional spending on new health care facilities and services had a positive "policy image."[5] The popularity of programs such as the Hill-Burton Act of 1946, the dramatic growth of private health insurance plans, and the expansion of the Veterans Administration hospital system reflected the support of policymakers and the public for expanding access to health care. By the late 1960s, however, policymakers increasingly viewed health care spending as a problem rather than an opportunity. As state governments became significant purchasers of health care, additional spending on Medicaid and employee health benefits was seen less as an "investment" in extending needed services to the poor and underserved than as a "crisis" that raised the specter of budget deficits, program cutbacks, and higher taxes. To cope with these new fiscal pressures, public officials in many states embarked upon a "government-led search for solutions to government's problems" (Brown 1982, 45) in an effort to control the rapidly rising costs of open-ended entitlement programs.

The health care cost crisis manifested itself in two distinct ways at the state level over the past two decades. Health care costs have both a direct and an indirect impact on the fiscal health of state governments. The most direct impact of rising health care costs was seen in the growth of state Medicaid expenditures, which emerged as "budget busters" in many states during the tight fiscal climate of the late 1980s and early 1990s (Gold 1994). In part, rising state Medicaid expenditures were the result of intentional policy choices by state governments that allowed states to shift the costs of state human services programs to Medicaid in order to qualify for federal matching funds. Other states imposed provider taxes or encouraged providers to donate free care services in order to qualify for higher disproportionate share hospital funds (Coughlin et al. 1994). The end result of these policies, however, was a rapid increase in state Medicaid spending during the early 1990s. Continued health care inflation in the Medicaid program, along with the rising cost of health insurance benefits for state workers, thus constituted a significant fiscal burden for state governments by the early 1990s, particularly in states with generous Medicaid programs that offered either expanded eligibility for the medically needy or optional services.

Rising health care costs also created an indirect fiscal problem for state policymakers, for they threatened the ability of states to attract and retain business investment and jobs. By the mid 1980s, states were actively engaged in a bidding war to attract new industry. Health care costs, however, were a growing problem for businesses, for they represented a highly unpredictable and expensive component of firms' labor costs. While states traditionally sought to woo businesses with tax breaks, investment incentives, and job training funds (Brace 1995), policymakers in states with higher than average health care costs feared that unless the cost of employee fringe benefits stabilized, established firms would leave for more hospitable business climates or refuse to invest in new jobs and facilities. Furthermore, state efforts to lure new businesses were also jeopardized by health care cost inflation, for while most state incentives were short-lived or targeted capital expenditures, health insurance and worker's compensation insurance represented an ongoing burden for new companies.

State policymakers, particularly those seeking elective office, thus had a powerful incentive to control health care costs over the past two decades. In a fiscal climate defined by sharp reductions in intergovernmental aid and new federal mandates, states could no longer turn to the federal government for solutions to their budgetary problems. In the aftermath of the property tax revolt of the late 1970s, many states also sought to increase revenue sharing and other aid to local governments in order to provide property tax relief. In this context, rationalizing policies aimed at controlling rampant inflation in the health sector had a powerful appeal for policymakers. Higher taxes or an inability to attract and retain businesses and jobs represented a serious threat to officeholders intent on winning reelection. Since public officials must be concerned with reelection regardless of their goals or motivations (Arnold 1990; Fiorina 1990; Mayhew 1974), challenging the autonomy of providers is not as irrational as it first appears.

The success of state officials in expanding their administrative capabilities and control over the hospital industry supports Higgs' (1987) contention that crisis, either perceived or real, is a precondition for the expansion of government authority. Few studies of state politics and policy-making, however, have explored the role of crisis in structuring policy change (Stonecash 1996). This is a particularly significant omission in the literature on state health care policy, where the rhetoric of crisis has defined the terms of policy debate for more than two decades. Crises, whether perceived or real, can break down ideological and interest group opposition to the use of public authority. The urgency of states' fiscal problems frequently led policymakers to embrace policies which challenged the professional sovereignty and fiscal autonomy of health care providers. As a result, policies which would have been unthinkable in the past—from the development of elaborate rate-setting methodologies to limitations on the capital investments and services of hospitals—were commonplace by the early 1980s (Brown 1986). The expansion of state power over the health care industry, however, largely emerged from technical alterations of the prevailing reimbursement methodology, not through extended public debate. This experience offers an important lesson in how states respond to emerging policy problems, for the process of state-building, in which public officials create new political institutions and develop the problem-solving capacities of existing government agencies, may proceed far from the public eye in policy arenas where mastery of a body of specialized knowledge is a prerequisite for participation in policy debates.[6]

REGIMES AND THE POLICY PROCESS

Current policy dilemmas are often the product of prior actions, unfounded assumptions, or difficulties in program implementation, for the design of regulatory institutions and the unintended consequences of prior policy choices continue to shape regulatory outcomes in later years (Heclo 1974; Skocpol 1993). Malcolm Jewell (1982, 653) underscores the need to "develop a theoretical perspective that will help us to identify the forces that distinguish one state from another and to explain how states change or resist the pressures for change." To date, few studies of health care regulation have examined the consequences of different institutional forms or the long-term impact of state-building on policy choices and implementation.[7] This is unfortunate, for contemporary debates occur in the shadows of the rules and limits of existing political institutions, the long-standing relationships and tensions among participants in the regulatory process, and the larger political culture of a state (Skowronek 1982; Skocpol 1985).

Successful state cost-containment programs, therefore, do not depend exclusively on whether providers are reimbursed by a single payer or multiple payers; paid prospectively or retrospectively; or whether reimbursement is computed on a per diem, per case, or global budget basis. As Foster (1982) notes, the rate of reimbursement can be set at a high or low level under any payment methodology. Cost control is inextricably linked to the capacity and autonomy of regulatory institutions, for without adequate authority and expertise, public officials will be hard pressed to design and implement an effective health care financing system.

Differences in policy choices, program implementation, and programmatic outcomes among states appear less perplexing if one conceives of the policy-making environment in a state as a distinctive policy regime. Unlike regulatory issue networks (Gormley 1986) or policy subsystems (Meier 1985), policy regimes encompass not only the groups and issue entrepreneurs engaged in policy-making, but also the institutions, rules, and norms which shape policy formation, decision-making and implementation on a given issue (see Krasner 1983). Regimes are particularly useful as an organizing principle for studying regulatory politics because they situate the behavior of relevant actors in the larger institutional and ideological environment in which they operate. A regime, however, is not simply a collection of political organizations operating within a particular policy subsystem or issue network. Instead, regimes govern the actions of their members by defining "patterns of behavior or practice around which expectations converge" (Young 1983, 93). As social institutions, regulatory regimes exhibit identifiable patterns, or regularities, in the behavior of their participants that endure over time. Furthermore, behavior under any given regime may either be self-policed or specified by rules issued by government or another external authority (Schotter 1988).

Each of the cases described below suggests that a state's efforts to control health care costs are shaped by the nature of its prevailing regulatory regime. Different regimes offer alternative paths to controlling health care costs, for the design and capacity of state regulatory institutions, as well as the relationship between state officials and the regulated industry, will affect a state's ability to create and maintain an effective system of regulation. Although regulatory regimes reflect the larger policy-making environment in a state, regulatory politics may look quite different from industry to industry and over time, depending on the salience of the issue to the mass public (Gormley 1986; Meier 1985), the policy image associated with the issue, its relevance to key policymakers, and the organization and cohesion of industry groups and other societal interests. Furthermore, regimes vary according to whether essential decisions about the organization, financing, and delivery of health care services are made by the state, by societal groups, or through a partnership between state officials and affected interests.[8] The classification of regulatory regimes, therefore, depends on the answer to a basic question about the relationship between state officials and societal groups: To what extent are decisions by organizations directed or controlled by the actions of the state?

Different regulatory regimes reflect fundamental differences in (1) the nature of the decision-making and implementation process and (2) the ability of state agencies to change the behavior of health care providers. As Migdal (1988, 31) observed, "the most subtle and fascinating patterns of political change and political inertia have resulted from the accommodation between states and other powerful organizations in society." While the range of participants in health care policy-making does not vary considerably from one state to the next, the relationships among state officials and private interests will change from one regime to another. In some states, interest groups will be active participants in developing and implementing policy choices; in others, opportunities for participation by groups are limited to testifying at hearings and lobbying decision makers. The effectiveness of state cost-control programs, however, is a function of the state's capability to "plan and transform" the industry (Migdal 1988) through either incentives or controls. The potential and capability of a state's regulatory apparatus is rarely constant. Instead, the relative importance of regulation as a cost-control strategy and the state's capacities to implement such an approach changes in response to shifting political, ideological, and economic trends.

The relationship between state governments and the hospital industry falls into three distinct patterns, or regimes, which are biased either in favor of or against the development of regulatory solutions to control hospital costs (Hackey 1992). Each regime represents a fundamentally different balance between the "relative bargaining strengths of purchasers and providers" (Thorpe 1993, 479). At one extreme, *imposed regimes* are defined by an extreme centralization of state regulatory powers, where public officials possess the authority to reshape the hospital reimbursement process to further the state's interests. In contrast, *market regimes* are notable for the relative underdevelopment of state regulatory authority and the delegation of public authority to private groups. Under *negotiated regimes,* a recurring tension over the proper means and ends of state regulation remains unresolved, leading to shifting relationships among providers, payers, and public officials.

The prevailing method of reimbursement does not determine the nature of a state's hospital regulatory regime. Instead, the role of the state in shaping the organizational behavior of health care providers and the degree to which providers comply with and participate in the regulatory process determines whether a state's approach to hospital cost containment falls under a particular regime. Each regime, however, reflects not only the extent of state regulation and the capacities of the state, but a fundamentally different relationship between state and society (Gilbert and Howe 1991). While state intervention is greatest under an imposed regime, state authority is not absent under a market regime, for as Migdal (1988, 16) notes, "if there are those who still do not play by the market's rules, the state will use its authority to enforce contracts made in the marketplace." In addition to the scope of state regulatory powers, therefore, the process of interest group intermediation and the legitimacy of state intervention are central to the definition of a regulatory regime.

Imposed Regimes

Health care policy-making under an imposed regulatory regime is characterized by an authoritative decision-making process which structures the behavior of health care providers and third-party payers. Public officials extend their control over private groups through a combination of rules, regulations, and incentives which affect the management decisions of providers and third-party payers. Regulatory powers, furthermore, are consolidated within institutions defined and controlled by the state; while public officials regularly consult with industry groups under an imposed regulatory regime, the locus of decision-making remains centralized within the institutions of state government. As a result, imposed regimes are characterized by a high degree of autonomy on the part of public officials; the state is able to pursue its agenda despite opposition from powerful societal groups (Prechel 1990). The resulting policy-making environment supports an extensive role for public officials in determining the form and level of reimbursement for health care providers and the circumstances under which hospitals and other providers may add or modify their existing services.

In general, policymakers in states governed by imposed regulatory regimes favor an authoritative approach to controlling health care costs, improving access to health services, and maintaining the quality of care. As a result, the decision-making and implementation process under imposed regimes is often the target of intense criticism from the regulated industry. State officials, however, possess sufficient political resources to protect the state's expanded regulatory role despite recurring conflicts with industry groups. The ability of state policymakers to preserve a centralized regulatory apparatus, however, is contingent upon the scope of the state's statutory mandate to regulate health care providers, the capacity of state political institutions, and the cohesiveness of state policymakers within the health care-issue network.

Imposed regulatory regimes are defined by a broad statutory mandate that permits state officials to claim jurisdiction over critical areas of hospital reimbursement and management. In addition to the breadth of state regulatory powers, imposed regimes endow policymakers with considerable rule-making powers to implement their statutory mandate. The state's regulatory strategy, in short, is both coordinated and cohesive, as policymakers collaborate to achieve shared goals. As a result, the interests and actions of the state may be described as a coherent unit, in which conflicts among agencies and policymakers responsible for implementing policy are the exception, not the rule.

A high degree of policy cohesion (Robertson 1993), however, requires strong leadership and political support. Imposed regimes are highly institutionalized; policy-making is centralized within, and defined by, professionalized state agencies.* The central role of state agencies in setting policy facilitates the recruitment and retention of well-educated professionals to career civil service positions in state government. In part, the unity of purpose characteristic of imposed regimes stems from the long tenure of senior policymakers, who bring an extensive "institutional memory" to policy debates. Political appointees, furthermore, are rarely inclined to challenge the prerogatives of senior careerists whose advice and expertise are crucial to managing the state's regulatory apparatus.

State officials may carry out their broad statutory mandate to control costs through a variety of cost-control strategies which are designed, coordinated, or implemented by state bureaucratic agencies. An imposed regime, however, is not defined by a commitment to a particular cost-containment strategy (e.g., rate setting). Regardless of the payment methodology, however, hospital reimbursement and investment are guided, if not directly controlled by, state regulatory institutions. These decisions, furthermore, are consonant with the interests of the state, rather than those of private groups in the issue network.

The authoritative nature of state policy-making under imposed regulatory regimes leads to repeated and often intense conflicts between state officials and industry representatives. Private groups in the issue network are seldom granted formal incorporation into the decision-making or implementation process. As a result, providers, payers, and other interested parties are reactive, rather than proactive, participants in policy debates. Policy options are formulated by public officials in the legislature or the executive branch to achieve the state's goals; while interest groups are active participants in legislative debates and administrative rule-making, they do not define the content of the public agenda. In an imposed regime, the "balance of power" in the issue network lies in the public sector. While conflict over both the scope and substance of state regulatory powers often pervades imposed regimes, on most issues public officials possess the administrative expertise and political support to achieve their ends.

Imposed regimes, in sum, are defined by the presence of coercive state authority. Policy-making on matters of substance is directed or coordinated by state agencies in pursuit of the state's interests. The presence of highly professionalized and differentiated policy-making institutions provides the state with the "essential tentacles" (Migdal 1988) needed to enforce compliance with its goals. While the state may seek to achieve its ends through either rules or incentives, essential decisions about the rate of payment, the utilization of health care services, and the introduction of new technologies are determined through a public process designed and controlled by the state.

Negotiated Regimes

In many states, public officials lack the resources or the political support to impose regulatory solutions upon a recalcitrant industry. When public officials are unable to impose regulation on the industry, they may nevertheless be able to negotiate a partnership with societal interests to achieve their goals. The creation of negotiated regimes, therefore, involves the active participation of industry groups and other interested parties in designing, implementing, and administering regulatory policy choices. The choice of policy instruments under negotiated regimes and the scope of the state's statutory mandate emerge as products of mutual accommodation. Negotiated regimes do not preclude coercive policy instruments such as rate-setting or global budgets, but in contrast to imposed regimes, such arrangements typically require the consent of, if not active collaboration with, private groups within the issue network. As a result, the regulatory process is often less conflictual than imposed regimes, for the institutional framework and/or the extent of the state's role are the product of extensive bargaining between public and private interests.

The necessity of building a consensus among public and private decision makers also is reflected in the design of state cost-containment initiatives. Under negotiated regimes, participation in many cost-containment initiatives is voluntary; while such arrangements can often yield considerable cost savings (e.g., by establishing purchasing cooperatives or targets for expenditure growth), voluntary programs lack the ability to sanction noncompliant groups. Since negotiated regimes are based upon the active participation, if not incorporation, of industry groups in the regulatory process, many of the functions normally performed by the state under imposed regimes may be delegated to private or quasi-public groups. The ability of state policymakers to plan and implement cost-control initiatives without assistance from private groups (e.g., the state hospital association or third-party insurers) is limited. Furthermore, proposals to grant new authority and oversight capabilities to the state without a provision for participation and input from the regulated industry will be regarded as unnecessary or threatening to the interests of private groups.

Although negotiated regimes are based upon mutual consent, the balance of power between state and society is often tenuous. While participants may be able to reach agreement concerning the form of reimbursement or the degree of state oversight, lingering disputes about the proper role of the state and the scope of its regulatory powers often lurk beneath the surface of policy debates in a negotiated regime. Changes in medical practice, economic conditions, or the introduction of new health care delivery systems may destabilize a fragile consensus among public and private decision makers and undermine the state's authority to control pricing and allocation decisions. If participant interests change over time, the negotiated agreement that binds the parties in the regulatory process together may come apart at the seams. Unless a new round of negotiations between legislators, executive branch policymakers, and societal groups is able to forge a new consensus, dissatisfied groups may push to weaken or repeal the existing system of regulatory controls.

Market Regimes

Market regimes reflect an enduring belief in the ability of competition to resolve difficult questions of cost and the efficient allocation of institutional resources. Decision-making and implementation rest in the hands of private groups (e.g., payers, providers, businesses) under a market regime, with little coordination or regulation by the state. The choice of instruments to control costs—prospective or retrospective payment mechanisms, limits on the acquisition and utilization of new technologies, and the level of reimbursement—are determined through the interaction of private groups. Some government oversight of hospitals will occur in every state; market regimes, however, are characterized by a minimal level of state involvement in the internal affairs of the hospital industry.[9] Since the principal locus of activity lies in the private sector, state agencies responsible for administering certificate-of-need or other regulatory programs will find it difficult to recruit and retain professional staff. In the absence of strong budgetary support and a clear statutory mandate, regulatory agencies under market regimes seldom emerge as incubators of innovative new policies. Similarly, state agencies are less differentiated than their counterparts in other regimes, for most specialized activities related to provider payment are managed by private groups or trade associations (e.g., the state hospital association).

In states where the hospital industry is governed by a market regime, however, state involvement will be limited to those areas which are either mandated by federal guidelines or which are necessary to protect the health and safety of the public (e.g., basic operating standards). Where policymakers and the public espouse a firm belief in the efficacy of market competition, the role of government in regulating health care providers will be limited to ensuring that providers and payers do not engage in anticompetitive practices and that the safety of consumers and patients is protected.[10]

The limited role of state officials is also reflected in a weak, or largely symbolic, statutory mandate that confers few regulatory powers on state agencies to monitor industry performance, oversee new construction, and influence the decisions of hospital administrators. From the perspective of public officials, health care providers, and the public, however, the absence of significant coercive state power is not a shortcoming in a market regime. In this view, government regulation of prices, capital projects, and other issues related to the management and organization of hospital services have the potential to distort market forces by protecting inefficient producers or keeping prices artificially high by protecting hospitals from competition. Instead, policymakers in market regimes are likely to embrace Schultze's (1977, 7) notion that regulation and other forms of social intervention "ought to maximize the use of techniques that modify the structure of private incentives rather than those that rely on the command-and-control approach of centralized bureaucracies."

Market regimes are defined by a basic consensus among participants about the role of the state. While providers often disagree with state officials about the adequacy of Medicaid reimbursement or the application of new standards for the inspection of clinical laboratories, conflicts between the state and other participants in the state's health care policy-issue network are sporadic, not sustained. The relative quiescence of health care policy-making under market regimes is closely tied to the lack of state involvement in the daily affairs of health care providers; with little at stake, private groups have little to fear from public officials. Under these circumstances, autonomous action by the state is seldom possible; state officials lack the statutory authority and the legitimacy needed to support significant extensions of governmental power over the hospital industry.[11] Market regimes are most likely to endure in states where public officials lack a significant justification for intervening in the affairs of the regulated industry (e.g., in states where Medicaid spending consumes a relatively low proportion of the state budget).

The consensual nature of health care policy-making under market regimes also reflects the state's prevailing political culture, which emphasizes the virtues of private solutions to public problems (McConnell 1966). In the context of a firm belief in the ability of market competition to generate socially optimal outcomes, state intervention is unnecessary. Even if the policy image associated with health care costs in general, and hospital spending in particular, emphasizes the importance of controlling costs, state regulation of the hospital industry faces a crisis of legitimacy in a market regime. In this environment, policymakers and the public are likely to regard more effective competition, rather than government controls, as the solution to the state's health care cost crisis.

THE FUTURE OF STATE HEALTH CARE REGULATION

Society does not face a stark choice between two polar opposites of competition and regulation, for the actions of government officials structure the operation of the marketplace (Morone 1992). The state need not intervene directly in the operation of the private sector to have a significant impact on policy outcomes; its role in establishing the rules that govern market activities ensures that to some extent policy always reflects the preferences of state officials. Investigating the form of state intervention is more profitable than focusing on the level of state activity in the economy. Each of the regimes described above represents a distinctive approach to decision-making among public and private actors within a policy subsystem. On a basic level, the role of the state in setting priorities, making decisions, and administering policy leads to fundamental differences among regimes in different states. These differences, in turn, reflect the presence of divergent values and interests among public and private actors in health care policy-making.

Government can be extensively involved in a limited range of policy areas or have superficial involvement in many different policy arenas, but the scope of activity, in and of itself, tells only part of the story about the relationship between government and society. Public officials face a choice of potential strategies ranging from outright government ownership or direct regulation of the industry to the delegation of regulatory powers to industry groups. In many circumstances, public officials opt for a market-based strategy, even when the possibility of public action is not proscribed (Barrow 1993a). Thus, "differences in the balance of market and government activity are not themselves indications of the strength or weakness of the state or of private enterprise" (Ikenberry 1988, 45).

Subsequent chapters develop and apply the framework introduced in this chapter to explain *why* states followed the paths that they did to control health care costs. Past state efforts to control health care costs can shed light on the problems and prospects of contemporary plans to reshape the health care system. In particular, state experiences with rate setting and certificate-of-need regulation illustrate the essential characteristics of state health care policy-issue networks. In the wake of recent proposals to transform Medicaid into a block grant to the states and the ongoing popularity of state waiver programs, understanding the political dynamics of health care policy-making at the state level in the 1990s takes on renewed importance.

Furthermore, the discussion of the administrative capacity and policy-making expertise of state governments in each of the states analyzed below is particularly relevant for students of contemporary health care policy-making. Ironically, while state regulation of health care providers has changed over the past decade, the dramatic growth of managed care has brought new demands for state regulation of health care providers and third-party payers. The nature of regulation has changed from traditional price and entry regulation to an emphasis on outcomes assessment and quality assurance. In particular, a diverse coalition of consumers and businesses has petitioned state legislatures to take steps to mitigate the detrimental effects of unrestricted market competition among health insurers and providers by mandating minimum hospital stays and establishing "report cards" that rate the performance of physicians and hospitals. This new regulatory environment presents fresh challenges for state regulators, who must now struggle to define and monitor the quality of patient care; assemble data on quality, price, and outcomes for individual "consumers" and businesses; and ensure that increased competition among health care providers does not threaten the viability of the existing patchwork system for financing care for the poor and uninsured.

State health care policy-making remains in a state of flux. While many states have deregulated their hospital payment systems in recent years, others developed new policy tools to influence the behavior of health care providers and third-party payers. The next chapter explores the circumstances under which policy regimes change in an effort to develop an evolutionary approach to the study of regulatory policy. Theories of state policy-making must explain both variation across states and over time within states. By examining the institutional and ideological underpinnings of state policy regimes along with the patterns of interest group intermediation, Chapter 2 develops hypotheses to account for regime transformation (e.g., deregulation).

Chapters 3 through 6 apply the regime framework to a comparative case study of health care policy-making in New York, Massachusetts, Rhode Island, and New Hampshire over the past three decades. Each chapter describes the nature of the state's prevailing policy regime in the 1990s and discusses its political evolution and future prospects. Since all four states have recently received Medicaid waivers, the case studies also afford an opportunity to examine how pro-competitive policies (e.g., Medicaid managed care programs) can be integrated within existing state cost-containment programs. The cases also permit a detailed comparison of the effectiveness of competitive versus regulatory approaches to controlling hospital costs. The final chapter highlights the problems and prospects facing state efforts to control health care costs in the years ahead, drawing upon lessons learned from each of the cases discussed below.

CHAPTER NOTES

1. A 1992 decision by the New Jersey Supreme Court that invalidated the state's reimbursement methodology as a violation of the 1974 Employee Retirement and Income Security Act, however, forced the state to restructure its entire hospital financing system. For a more detailed discussion of this

issue, see Chirba-Martin and Brennan's (1994) excellent discussion of ERISA's importance to state health care reform and cost-containment initiatives.

2. Even in the absence of a capital cap, however, a singular focus on the rate of project denials or the savings in capital and operating costs associated with rejected CON applications understates the impact of capital expenditure controls on providers' behavior. Since the deliberations which accompany the CON review process often lead to concessions by providers, modifications of proposed projects offer a viable alternative to achieving regulators' desired objectives (e.g., expanding care for the uninsured, lowering operating costs by requiring a higher equity contribution by applicants). Furthermore, as Tierney, Waters, and Rosenberg (1982) argue, effective communication between state regulatory agencies and providers should minimize the number of denials. The existence of CON may also deter providers from submitting weak proposals for review, for "few institutions are likely to expend the time, energy, and money to traverse the complex certificate-of-need process for a project that cannot withstand the test of public scrutiny" (Tierney, Waters, and Rosenberg 1982, 178).

3. Arizona was the only state which elected to not participate in the Medicaid program; responsibility for financing health care for the poor was left in the hands of county governments in Arizona until 1982. For a more detailed account of the political origins of the Arizona Health Care Cost Containment System, see Brecher (1984).

4. New Jersey's early experience with all-payer rate-setting using diagnosis-related groups (DRGs) has been the basis for extensive generalization about the operation and effectiveness of regulation as a cost-control strategy, with few attempts to compare its experience to similar programs in other states. See Morone and Dunham (1983), Dunham and Morone (1984), and Widman and Light (1988) for an excellent description of the political evolution and implementation of rate regulation in New Jersey.

5. See Baumgartner and Jones' (1991) discussion of policy images and their impact on policy formulation.

6. Cobb and Elder (1983, 99–100) offer a useful discussion of the effects of complexity on issue expansion.

7. Jim Morone's (1990a) analysis of the evolution of contemporary health care policy constitutes a significant exception to this point.

8. As Lawson (1993, 187) notes, a regime "has less to do with power per se than the way in which power is actually used. A regime, then, may be characterized as that part of the political system which determines how and under what conditions and limitations the power of the state is exercised."

9. Current federal practice necessitates that state health departments oversee the quality of care provided by doctors and hospitals serving Medicare and Medicaid patients; state officials also have a dual role as both regulators and purchasers for state Medicaid programs.

10. While Milton Friedman (1980) and other conservative thinkers have argued for the abolition of state licensing requirements for medical providers as an unnecessary interference on the operation of free markets, few contemporary proposals for market-based reform seek such sweeping changes. The most

sweeping proposal for market-based reform in the 103rd Congress was the Consumer Choice Health Security Act proposed by Sen. Don Nickels (R-OK) and Rep. Clifford Stearns (R-FL). Under the Nickels-Stearns plan, individuals would be given powerful tax incentives to purchase health insurance coverage; the overall structure of the plan was based upon the Federal Employees Health Benefits Program (FEHBP), which allows employees to choose from a range of competing health plans. The core assumption of this plan and of similar proposals for market reform is that consumers will shop on the basis of price for health insurance if they are required to shoulder the burden of financing their own coverage rather than having its cost subsidized by their employers or the government (e.g., through Medicare, Medicaid).

11. Using Nordlinger's (1981) description of "Type III" state autonomy, the state may achieve its ends in areas where the preferences of public officials and private groups do not diverge. In the absence of consensus over the direction of policy, however, state officials are generally unable to persuade societal groups to adopt its preferences or to enact policies opposed by significant economic or political interests.

2

Stability and Change in Policy Regimes

By the early 1990s, health care policy-making had become unpredictable and chaotic in many states. As legislators, interest groups, and bureaucrats scrambled to control Medicaid spending, expand access to the uninsured, and prop up ailing urban hospitals, constant change, rather than stability, characterized the era. In the short span of five years, several states that had been early leaders in regulating the hospital industry abandoned or significantly weakened their rate-setting and certificate-of-need programs. After 1990, Connecticut, Maine, Massachusetts, Minnesota, New Jersey, and New York deregulated their hospital payment systems in favor of market-based competition (McDonough 1995). Other states that had never challenged the prerogatives of health care providers sought to reinvent their health care delivery systems. In 1993 and 1994, all-payer or single-payer financing systems were seriously debated in Minnesota, Montana, and Vermont. Numerous state reform commissions considered a wide range of regulatory strategies to control health care costs after the demise of the Clinton administration's Health Security Act in 1994.

These developments raise several important, yet often unasked, questions about state health care policy-making. In particular, analyses of contemporary health care policy must be able to account for both continuity and change in state policy subsystems. The flurry of change in recent years underscores the importance of understanding how policy regimes form and evolve over time. In addition, the growing popularity of deregulation as a cost-control strategy poses new challenges for models of the policy process; pinpointing the factors which contribute to the transformation or dissolution of existing regimes is essential. Why are patterns of policy-making stable in some regimes yet unstable in others? This chapter develops a model of regime change to explain the evolution of state health care policy-making.

CONTEMPORARY EXPLANATIONS OF POLICY CHANGE

Contemporary health care policy-making casts doubts upon the notion that the winners and losers in regulatory politics are largely determined by which groups have the strongest incentives to become politically active (Wilson 1980). The composition of state health policy subsystems tells little about which groups will prevail in policy debates over alternative cost containment. Strategies for state health care policy-issue networks—business groups, health providers, third party insurers, and state officials—are remarkably similar from state to state. The involvement of public interest groups and the public in health care financing issues is both limited and sporadic due to the complex and highly technical nature of most policy debates.[1] As a result, differences in the relative influence of participants within issue networks and the relationship between affected interests and state officials have emerged as critical factors in explaining the wide variation in state policy choices.

In addition, health care policy-making is played out in different institutional settings. The success or failure of state regulatory programs depends on whether decision-making authority lies within the legislature, the executive branch, or independent regulatory agencies. Unlike regulation in other policy domains, the "consumers" who purchase health care services are typically well-organized, active participants in the policy-making process. Over the past two decades, insurers, business, and state government agencies have joined hospitals and other health care providers at the bargaining table to draft legislation on health care regulation and financing (Martin 1993; Brown 1993). Due to these changes in the policy-making environment, existing models of state health care policy-making fall short in explaining the recent upheavals in health care financing and regulation over the past decade.

Capture

The study of regulatory behavior remains in a state of flux after more than a decade of sweeping changes in the relationship of state governments with several of the nation's largest industries. Prior to the 1980s, prevailing models painted a picture of regulation as a process dominated by powerful societal interests. The politics of the regulatory process, it was often noted, reflected the concerns of the well-organized and well-funded industry lobbies (Kolko 1965), many of which were populated with former government employees who had left their federal jobs for higher pay, better hours, and better working conditions in the private sector (Sapolsky, Aisenberg, and Morone 1987). Although most explanations of regulatory politics concurred that client groups or regulated industries often "captured" their would-be regulators, scholars disagreed over how to explain these recurring patterns of industry dominance.

Early accounts of regulatory capture emphasized the effects of natural changes in an agency's "life cycle" on the relationships of regulatory agencies with client groups (Bernstein 1955). Economic theories of regulatory failure held that regulation was typically "acquired by the industry and . . . designed and operated primarily for its benefit" (Stigler 1988), while others suggested that the design of the regulatory process had inadvertently tilted the balance of power in favor of industry groups by fragmenting public authority among a multitude of specialized regulatory bodies (McConnell 1966) or through excessive delegation of policy-making responsibilities to unelected representatives (Lowi 1969). As James Q. Wilson (1973) argued, industry capture of regulatory agencies was likely when government policies "confer concentrated benefits on a small, organizable segment of society and impose only widely distributed costs on a large, hard-to-organize segment of society."

The advent of new forms of social regulation and the deregulation of several of the nation's largest industries underscored the inadequacy of theories that viewed government regulatory agencies as prisoners of narrowly based functional constituencies. Nontraditional forms of regulation, typified by the rise of the consumer protection movement, occupational safety and health legislation, and a wide range of environmental regulations, gradually gained prominence over traditional price-and-entry regulations during the 1960s and 1970s (Meier 1985). These new programs were neither demanded by the private sector to minimize destructive competition nor (in most cases) dominated by industry groups (Derthick and Quirk 1985). Cases in which regulation has been imposed on an industry against its will, as in health care, or where deregulation occurs over the protests of the regulated industry, constitute exceptions to society-centered explanations. Indeed, the fundamental weakness of pluralist models of regulatory capture is their narrow focus on interest groups as the agents of policy change.[2]

When applied to state health policy-making, pluralist explanations—such as Mindy Widman and Donald Light's (1988) examination of New Jersey's experience with hospital rate regulation—greatly underestimate the autonomy of state officials. In Widman and Light's view, changes in New Jersey's approach to regulating the state's hospital industry emerged in response to the hospitals' plea for government intervention and the acquiescence of third-party insurers and other key interest groups. Their analysis concluded that health care providers can effectively limit the scope of regulation and/or receive compensatory damages in return for their political support of an independent regulatory commission to oversee the payment process (Widman and Light 1988, 9). Such a conclusion, however, significantly understates the critical role of state officials within the New Jersey Department of Health in expanding the scope of the payment system (Morone and Dunham 1984). While third-party payers and health care providers dominated the initial efforts at regulating hospital rates and facilities construction in New Jersey, by the late 1970s the state had reclaimed the authority it previously ceded to the hospital industry (Morone and Dunham 1985). Under the state's all-payer rate-setting methodology, state officials used their legislative mandate to regulate hospital rates, thereby completely controlling the industry's revenue stream.

Health care policy-making in New York and Massachusetts also fails to conform to the expectations of traditional pluralist models of regulatory politics. Under the leadership of Commissioner David Axelrod, the New York Department of Health successfully implemented a highly restrictive payment system for inpatient hospital care in New York during the 1970s and 1980s despite howls of protest from the hospital industry (Hackey 1992). In Massachusetts, state officials entered into an active partnership with business and industry groups to create an all-payer rate-setting system in the early 1980s (Bergthold 1988; 1990b). In neither case were state officials "captured" by the hospital industry. Far from acting as impartial mediators of group conflict, state agencies led efforts to reshape the health care financing system to serve broader public goals such as cost containment and expanded access to care for the uninsured. Cases such as Massachusetts, New Jersey, and New York expose a fundamental weakness of societal models of regulatory capture; a narrow focus on interest groups as the agents of policy change underestimates the role of public officials in setting the policy agenda and making independent policy choices.[3]

Corporatism

The technocratic nature of many health policy issues, coupled with the claims of health care providers on the issue of professional hegemony over the delivery of medical care, encourages extensive consultation with affected interests in making state health care policy. While few policy domains in the U.S. resemble the corporatist systems of interest group intermediation present in many European democracies, studies of state health and industrial policy (Bergthold 1988; Hudson, Hyde, and Carroll 1987; Gray and Lowery 1990; Tierney 1987) confirm that state governments often delegate public resources and powers to private groups through either formal or informal means. A defining characteristic of corporatist interest intermediation is the formal delegation, or sharing, of public authority with private interest groups (Brand 1988; Offe 1981).[4] Under corporatism, interest groups are "an integral part of administration; they are not merely consulted over the implementation of policy" (Cawson 1986).[5]

In a corporatist model, decisions are made by government only after extensive consultation and bargaining with affected industries. Over the past decade, health care policy-making in several states was held up as an example of corporatist bargaining and interest intermediation. In Massachusetts, private bargaining between business, health care providers, third-party payers, and state officials led to the creation of an all-payer rate-setting system in 1982. "The state initiated the participation of business in the policy process and allowed business to direct and make policy, and the state legislature ratified the decisions made by business and its private coalition" (Bergthold 1988, 448). By the mid-1980s, health care policy-making in New Jersey had also evolved into a meso-corporatist system in which affected interests were incorporated into the development and implementation of the state's uncompensated care trust fund (Brandon 1991). Under meso-corporatist bargaining, the state acts as an interest group, rather than an "impartial" actor, to further its own organizational and fiscal goals (Cawson 1986, Schmitter 1979).

Corporatist explanations of policy-making, however, assume that the various trade associations and professional groups possess the authority to bargain on behalf of their membership, for the policy-making process under meso-corporatism is limited to major sectoral interests (Cawson 1986). Since membership in state and national peak associations (e.g., trade organizations and professional groups) is seldom compulsory, such groups depend upon their members' continued goodwill and support for their influence. Corporatist accounts of health care politics ultimately falter at this point, for peak associations find it virtually impossible to command the loyalty of disaffected members who have the option of "freelancing" in order to strike a more amenable compromise with state officials. As a result, many peak associations are "weak" or "ineffectual" (Salisbury 1979), for industry groups seldom possess a representational monopoly over their membership.

Furthermore, the coalitions of businesses, health care providers, and state officials are often increasingly fragile; over time, conflicting interests among the participants may resurface, leading one or more of the parties to withdraw its support for the negotiated settlement produced by corporatist bargaining. Fiscal crisis at the state level, along with rising inequities in the state's uncompensated care pool, ultimately derailed the corporatist bargaining process in New Jersey by the early 1990s (Brandon 1991; Berliner and Delgado 1991). The corporatist period in Massachusetts ended in a similar fashion as business groups retreated from the bargaining table after the passage of the state's universal health insurance law in 1988 (Bergthold 1990a; Hackey 1992; Kronick 1990). In contrast, debates over comprehensive health care reform plans in Minnesota and Vermont involved closed-door bargaining among legislators rather than negotiations among peak associations and state officials over policy development and implementation (Leichter 1993a; 1993b). In short, corporatist policy-making arrangements are not absent from health care policy-making at the state level, but they are difficult to sustain in the face of changing political and economic circumstances.

The "Politics of Ideas"

The allure of market competition for state health policymakers over the past decade lends credence to the role of the "politics of ideas" (Derthick and Quirk 1985) in explaining the evolution of state cost-containment strategies. The growing popularity of competition reflects systemic changes in the organization and delivery of health care as well as growing dissatisfaction with existing regulatory controls. The appeal of competition and a corresponding belief that government regulatory programs were incapable of producing "efficient" outcomes had their origins within policy-making circles in the 1970s and 1980s. Spurred on by academics and professional think tanks, Derthick and Quirk (1985) claimed that the cause of deregulation was adopted by crucial policy entrepreneurs who actively campaigned for pro-competitive reforms. Still, evidence on the influence of the politics of ideas in state health care policy-making is mixed.

The rhetoric of competition during the Nixon and Reagan administrations signaled a new approach to controlling health care cost inflation. The influence of proponents of competition is apparent in the principal federal initiatives to control health care costs during this period, which encouraged enrollment in health maintenance organizations (HMOs) and the formation of business health care coalitions (Brown and McLaughlin 1990) as a means to increase price competition for health services. Until the early 1990s, however, competition never took hold in the health sector to the same extent that it did in other industries, outside of a few metropolitan areas and regions (e.g., Minneapolis-St. Paul).[6] Most pro-competitive reforms proposed during the 1970s and 1980s were never fully implemented, or in some cases, ever seriously entertained. Despite the growing popularity of free-market ideology, federal and state regulation of the hospital industry actually increased in both scope and intensity.

The deregulation of several state hospital rate-setting systems in the early 1990s affirms the importance of public ideas in shaping policy debates. The election of conservative Republican governors in Massachusetts, New Jersey, and New York in the early 1990s led to sweeping policy changes in each state. Each new administration regarded hospital rate-setting programs as a burdensome and unwarranted government intervention which stymied the operation of competitive markets. Similarly, the end of federal support for health planning in 1986 led twelve states to end certificate-of-need reviews of health care providers' capital projects (Mueller 1988; Burda 1991). The appeal of public ideas such as deregulation, however, varies from state to state and from time to time. Not all states that had embraced rate-setting or certificate-of-need controls abandoned their regulatory efforts in the face of critics' arguments. Furthermore, in several states the impetus to deregulate the hospital industry emerged in response to judicial challenges of existing rate-setting methodologies and financing mechanisms for uncompensated care. In particular, hospitals and insurers successfully challenged rate-setting systems in New Jersey and New York in state and federal courts on the grounds that both states had violated the provisions of the Employee Income and Retirement Security Act (ERISA) by forcing self-insured health plans to subsidize the cost of charity care and bad debt for all hospital patients. Although the U.S. Supreme Court ultimately upheld the right of states to regulate hospital rates for public purposes in 1995, the legal challenge forced state officials to develop alternative cost-containment strategies. In other states, state rate-setting programs were widely regarded as cumbersome, inflexible, or ineffective.

While the ideas of public officials and other policy entrepreneurs help to define the policy agenda, the "politics of ideas" occurs within each state's unique institutional and ideological climate. New ideas must be adopted by political elites with access to political resources to effect change (Higgs 1987). Thus, ideas which take root in some states may not find a receptive audience in others. The challenge for students of regulatory politics is to identify where and when new ideas are likely to take hold.

State autonomy

As major purchasers of care, state officials have acquired a strong interest in controlling health care costs. The desire to contain the cost of government entitlement programs has led public officials to embrace a "new style of politics" characterized by "a government-led search for solutions to [its] own problems" (Brown 1983 , 17–18). State governments now rival the federal government as the most salient actor for health care providers, as reimbursement issues are increasingly decided by state legislatures and specialized rate-setting agencies (e.g., the Health Care Financing Administration). As Tierney (1987, 115) argues, "the government's information, stakes, and preferences—in short, the government's interests—now increasingly define the interests of private groups, not the reverse."

A state-centered view of the policy-making process is the cornerstone of James Morone's discussion of federal and state cost-containment efforts over the past two decades. Morone and Dunham (1985) contend that entrepreneurial state officials in New Jersey exploited widespread cost shifting from regulated to unregulated payers and the fiscal difficulties of urban hospitals to wrest control of health care financing from health care providers. After the introduction of partial rate regulation in the mid-1970s, state officials used the promise of additional federal funding for uncompensated care under a Medicare demonstration waiver to persuade recalcitrant legislators and interest groups to implement a prospective all-payer reimbursement system using diagnosis-related groups (DRGs). Further, Morone and Dunham (1985, 272) claim that "once the program began to operate, it became difficult for interest groups to shape policy," for program development and implementation were dominated by professional bureaucrats within the New Jersey Department of Health.

In a similar vein, Morone (1990a) argued that local health planning programs stripped health care providers of their autonomy during the 1970s and early 1980s. By introducing lay people into health policy debates, local health systems agencies (HSAs) redefined the policy-making process at the state level by forcing providers to submit to an external review and planning process. Spurred on by federal officials to control costs, Morone argues that the membership and staff of HSAs embraced the goal of cost containment as a means of organizational preservation. The HSAs also provided a new institutional arena for decision-making, and offered new groups (e.g., businesses, unions, insurance companies) an opportunity to influence health policy for the first time. Health planning, however, was an unlikely candidate to wrest control of policy-making from providers, for it affected only a limited range of hospital activity. In addition, Sapolsky (1991a, 822) argues that "most hospital administrators quickly discovered that the planning system could be outmaneuvered. The system was not much of an obstacle once the consultants were called in to advise."

In short, a close examination of both the New Jersey experience and the legacy of federal and state health planning programs challenges the premise that contemporary health policy-making is dominated by professional state bureaucrats. While the Department of Health dominated decision-making on hospital reimbursement in New Jersey during the late 1970s and early 1980s, by the 1990s the Department had a more marginal role (Berliner and Delgado 1991). A high rate of personnel turnover, the loss of charismatic leadership, or persistent budgetary problems which constrain the ability of agencies to gather needed data and update regulatory controls to reflect a changing external environment may erode the influence of state officials in states where they once exercised substantial authority (Sapolsky, Aisenberg, and Morone 1987; Wilson 1989). The administrative capacity and policy-making autonomy of state officials are important elements of any model of state health care policy-making, but their importance fluctuates over time. State autonomy must be measured relative to the influence of private groups; states which are strong at one point in time may be weak at another (Barrow 1993a; Ikenberry 1988; Krasner 1978).

CHANGE AND CONTINUITY WITHIN POLICY REGIMES

Policy regimes are not static, but different regimes represent relatively stable and durable configurations of interests and institutions. To understand regime change, the set of "implicit or explicit principles, norms, rules, and decision-making procedures around which actors' expectations converge" (Krasner 1983, 2) must be identified. In a similar vein, Oran Young (1983, 93) notes that regime transformation results from changes in "recognized patterns of behavior or practice around which expectations converge." Every regime is rooted in a unique set of expectations about the nature of a given policy problem and assumptions about the proper role of government in forging solutions to such issues as rising health care costs and diminished access to health care. Fundamental changes in the expectations or interests of state and societal actors, therefore, are necessary conditions for regime transformation.

Regime dissolution or transformation is conceptually distinct from policy change *within* an existing regime. The former refers to a fundamental shift in values, expectations, and interests; the latter, to a consolidation or modification of existing power relationships. As Krasner (1983, 5) notes, "changes in rules and decision-making procedures are changes within regimes." Although the relationship between state government and private interests in a policy network changes over time, fluctuations in the administrative capacity or policy-making autonomy of public officials do not by themselves signal a regime change. The adoption of a new payment methodology for a state hospital rate-setting program, for example, would not signal a change of regime in a state which had previously regulated hospital rates. The introduction of regulatory controls into a state where decision-making on health care policy had previously been delegated to providers, however, represents a fundamental shift in the relationship between state and society. Similarly, the deregulation of hospital reimbursement or the cessation of capital expenditure controls also represents a basic shift in policy which redefines the relationship between state government and providers. In either case, new institutions or patterns of behavior supplant existing norms and rules which shape the process of decision-making and implementation.

As long as the basic expectations of actors and behavioral norms remain stable, changes in policy, decision-making, and shifting coalitions of interest groups will not precipitate a regime change (Krasner 1983). Policy innovations, conflicts, and recurring tensions among state and societal actors are in fact the normal practice of politics under imposed, negotiated, and market regimes. Conflict is present in all three regimes as groups and government officials struggle to define the policy agenda and determine "who gets what, when, and how" within the existing set of rules and behaviors established by the regime. Thus, short-term changes in the frequency or intensity of conflicts among affected interests, or between state and societal groups, may occur with regularity under any regime. The re-authorization of rate-setting controls or state funding for uncompensated care, for example, will often be accompanied by extensive lobbying and conflicts among businesses, health care providers, and third-party payers due to the economic stakes of such decisions for the relevant publics. Barring a dramatic shift in policy, however, relations between the actors in the regime will return to a state of "normal politics" after the negotiations and deliberations have concluded.

In a similar fashion, conflicts may also develop over representation on advisory councils or other policy-making bodies. In particular, the creation of new institutions such as purchasing alliances, local planning boards, or other cost-containment tools often leads to intense lobbying by providers, businesses, and other affected interests for seats on the governing boards or membership of the new organizations (Marmor and Morone 1981). The creation of hundreds of federally funded local health planning agencies in the 1970s led to intense competition for seats on the new health systems agencies, for "underlying the disputes about who should be represented was a debate about what the agencies ought to do" (Morone 1990a, 281).

Decisions about modifying the scope of state cost-containment programs often lead to heightened tension and conflict within a regime. The scope of the statutory authority of regulatory agencies delimits the range of policy alternatives for decision makers and defines the "rules of the game" for participants, effectively precluding some choices and favoring others (Skocpol 1993a). Hospital rate-setting programs which regulate only some third-party payers do not limit the ability of providers to shift costs to unregulated payers, ultimately weakening the ability of such states to control costs. Furthermore, unless capital expenditure controls apply to nonhospital providers, states will find it impossible to control systemwide health care costs, for physicians and hospitals will have an incentive to shift care to unregulated nonhospital settings such as freestanding surgical centers, dialysis centers, and diagnostic imaging facilities. By exempting certain groups from regulation (or conversely, incorporating previously unregulated providers or payers), policymakers advantage some participants at the expense of others.

Changes in the locus of decision-making authority are also commonplace within a policy regime. The locus of decision-making authority, or policy venue, within a regime structures the nature of the relationship between health care providers, third-party payers, and state officials. As Baumgartner and Jones (1991, 1047) note, "Each venue carries with it a decisional bias, because both participants and decision-making routines differ. When the venue of a public policy changes, as often occurs over time, those who previously dominated the policy process may find themselves in the minority, and erstwhile losers may be transformed into winners." Again, however, as long as the fundamental values and norms of participants do not change, administrative reorganizations will not alter the basic relationship between societal groups and the state. Different policy venues, however, can benefit some groups at the expense of others within a regime. Policy debates in the bureaucratic settings of independent commissions and executive agencies are more likely to focus on the interpretation of statutory requirements and the discretionary powers possessed by state officials than in legislative settings where issues are open to broader public participation and subject to extensive media coverage.

Similarly, the "coherence" of state policy-making agencies has powerful influence on policy choice and the prospects of successful program implementation within a regime. In this case, "coherence" represents the ability of policymakers to coordinate their activities and produce definitive and consistent policies (Robertson 1993). Conflict among various state agencies also determines the usefulness and appropriateness of referring to the state as a unitary actor for analytical purposes

(Ellis 1992). Where policy-making responsibilities have been delegated to more than one agency, opportunities arise for conflicts over strategies, resources, and the "ownership" of the issue (Rochefort and Cobb 1993). Problem ownership is critical to public officials, for agencies which exercise control over salient issues of concern to decision makers and the public are likely to attract and retain talented personnel and expand their claim on scarce resources. Conflicts over authority, strategies, and resources create opportunities for providers, insurers, and other societal actors to pit different government agencies against each other and may effectively impede the development of a coordinated cost-containment strategy.

In short, "regimes must be understood as something more than temporary arrangements that change with every shift of power or interests" (Krasner 1983, 2). Regimes are not static, but most conflicts *within* a regime are technical or procedural and do not challenge the underlying norms and principles which govern the behavior of participants. In states with well-established regulatory programs, conflicts will often arise over the interpretation of rules and statutory mandates, rather than the legitimacy or necessity of state intervention. In market regimes where decision-making authority has been ceded to private interests, tensions will emerge over which groups (e.g. providers or third-party payers) will shape and implement policy. In either case, participants are not seeking to change the basic values of the regime but rather are pursuing modifications to the implementation or administration of policy choices. Under these circumstances, debates are likely to revolve around the adequacy of payment, the timeliness of reimbursement, and delays in processing applications for review or updating payment schedules. When problems are regarded as technical in nature rather than as a conflict among opposing values, nonconflictual solutions can be devised through the application of professional expertise with limited public involvement and debate (May 1991, 194–96).

State authority over health care providers can erode over time in response to legal challenges or legislators' decisions to modify the scope of state regulatory powers or the nature of the regulatory process. As long as a fundamental consensus regarding the need for state involvement in some form remains, the underlying norms and patterns of policy-making within a state's policy regime remain intact. "If the principles, norms, rules, and decision-making procedures of a regime become less coherent, or if actual practice is inconsistent with principles, norms, rules, and procedures, then a regime has weakened" (Krasner 1983, 5). Even extensive modifications to a state's reimbursement methodology or CON program will not trigger a regime change if the basic structure of regulatory controls remains in place. Under these circumstances, conflict revolves around how the state will administer the programs in question, rather than around the legitimacy and appropriateness of state intervention.

In negotiated or imposed regimes, prolonged dissatisfaction with the hospital reimbursement process, for example, may be accompanied by increasingly contentious negotiations within the state legislature or by legal challenges to the state's implementation of its rate-setting mandate. Discontent with the process of capital expenditure review in many states was accompanied by calls by providers to shorten the length of the review process, modify the threshold or ceiling which triggers CON review, or exempt certain projects from review altogether. Under a market regime, conflicts among providers, third-party payers, and business groups over reimbursement and/or rising costs can produce new interest group alliances within an existing regime which shift the balance of power among societal groups. In recent years, third-party payers in several states have refused to contract with high-cost hospitals or sought to impose stringent new controls on providers, leading to intense conflict among physicians, hospitals, and third-party payers. Efforts by doctors and hospitals to enact "any willing provider" laws that would limit the ability of insurers to exclude providers from their networks have also contributed to growing tensions in state health care issue networks. An escalation of conflict within a regime, however, will not reshape the relationship between state and society unless the participants demand changes in the "principles and norms" of the regime itself (Krasner 1983).

UNDERSTANDING REGIME CHANGE

Left unresolved, sustained conflicts over the implementation of state policies or the functioning of private markets can erode popular support for a policy regime. In the case of state health care policy, regime change occurs when either the state or societal groups challenge the purpose or governance of a regime.[7] Regime changes occur through a two-stage process. The process of transformation begins with a catalyzing event or series of events that alter the distribution of costs and benefits among public and private actors. If efforts to patch the status quo fail, participants who are adversely affected by the new developments will seek to improve their circumstances either by withdrawing their support for the regime or by banding together with other disaffected groups in an effort to change the guiding principles of the regime. Catalysts of regime change may be either endogenous or exogenous. The former include emerging, or worsening, internal contradictions and the decisions of state courts; external agents of change include industrywide trends which affect the delivery of health care (e.g., the growth of managed care and secular declines in the length of hospital stays over the last decade) and new federal mandates or amendments to federal programs (e.g., Medicaid).

Catalysts of regime change strike at the principles and norms which undergird relationships among public officials and private groups. Thus, dissatisfaction with a particular decision or policy rarely leads to calls for dramatic shifts in the state's regulatory role. Instead, the transition period from one regime to another is characterized by a steady decline in what Easton (1975) terms "diffuse support." Applied to regulatory politics, diffuse support can be conceptualized as a belief in the legitimacy and efficacy of existing institutions and processes. Participants (particularly hospitals and third-party insurers) may disagree with individual decisions or specific policies yet still believe that the state has a role in regulating hospital reimbursement or capital projects in order to control costs and/or promote access to care. When participants begin to question the appropriateness or desirability of state regulation in any form, however, other changes in the policy environment may lead to a transformation of the existing regime.

The erosion of diffuse support for the regime's norms and principles creates an unstable policy-making environment. In the second stage of regime change, one or more intervening factors precipitate a regime transformation by fracturing existing alliances and forging new ones. The proximate causes, or precipitating factors, of regime change include (1) the development of a new ideological consensus among participants, (2) shifts in partisan control of state policy-making institutions, and (3) changes in the distribution of influence within the regime. Typically, however, regime transformation is precipitated by a confluence of factors, each weakening the political structure of alliances and interests which govern policy-making. The overall process of regime transformation is summarized in Table 2.1.

CATALYSTS OF REGIME CHANGE

Changes in one or more antecedent variables may serve as a catalyst for regime change by weakening support for existing institutional arrangements and behavioral norms. Four antecedent causes of regime change are discussed below: (1) fiscal crises and other internal contradictions; (2) changing patterns of health care financing and service delivery within the regime and the decisions of state courts; external agents of change include industrywide trends which affect the delivery of health care (e.g., the growth of managed care and secular declines in the length of hospital stays over the last decade); (3) policy changes

TABLE 2.1 The Process of Regime Transformation

Internal Contradictions	New Behavioral Norms and Values	Formation of a New Regime
Fiscal crises for state government pro-viders, or busi-nesses Changes in the health care delivery sys-tem (e.g., managed care) Intergovernmental mandates	Formation of new advo-cacy coalitions Shifting policy image of state policy tools Changing distribution of influence; incor-poration of new groups into the decision-making process	New "public philoso-phy" over the use of public authority New partisan and ideo-logical alignment Creation of new policy-making institu-tions Shift in the scope of state regulatory powers

at the federal level; and (4) the emergence of new policy images for existing or proposed policy instruments.

Internal Contradictions

By conferring benefits upon some groups and imposing costs upon others, all policy regimes create winners and losers. If the distribution of costs and benefits penalizes key participants, however, affected groups may withdraw their support for the regime and seek to establish a more favorable policy-making environment. As Young (1983, 107) observed, "Some regimes harbor internal contradictions that eventually lead to serious failures and mounting pressure for major alterations. Such contradictions may take the form of irreconcilable conflicts between central elements of a regime." Some internal contradictions may lie dormant for years and surface only in response to changing health care markets or patterns of care. Other policies, however, contain con-tradictions which are evident from their inception. In either case, inter-nal contradictions in policy design raise basic questions of equity among the principal partners in a regime and undermine its legitimacy in the eyes of providers, payers, or the state. In the absence of redistribu-tive " Band-Aids " to placate aggrieved parties, few regimes can with-stand a steady loss of support from key constituencies over time.

The evolution of health care financing in New Jersey over the past two decades offers a clear example of the role of internal contradictions in regime change. Legislators granted the state the power to review hospital rates in the early 1970s, but the state delegated responsibility for implementing the rate review process to the New Jersey hospital association; the NJHA, for its part, showed little interest in pursuing cost-containment by challenging the pricing practices of its members (Dunham and Morone 1983). By the mid-1970s, the state Department of Health reclaimed responsibility for the review process and promptly used its new authority to limit rate increases for Blue Cross and Medicaid. In response, hospitals simply shifted their charges to unregulated commercial insurers, whose rates increased dramatically in the wake of the state's decision to regulate the rates of some payers and not others. With few commercially insured patients, urban teaching hospitals found themselves in a fiscal crisis as a result of the state's decision to sharply reduce rate increases for Blue Cross and Medicaid. As Morone and Dunham (1985, 268) observed, "The new system of regulation was widely unpopular, marked by highly visible losers and few winners. Some hospitals approached bankruptcy, commercial health insurers suffered a severe competitive disadvantage, and for all the difficulties, medical inflation persisted because of cost-shifting."

In 1978 urban hospitals and commercial insurers responded to the growing fiscal crisis by embracing the state's proposal to regulate hospital rates for all payers. In addition to creating a state fund to finance the cost of uncompensated care, the new all-payer system limited the ability of hospitals to shift costs from regulated to unregulated payers and offered a lifeline to cash-strapped urban hospitals (Morone and Dunham 1985). In many ways, the uncompensated care fund was the glue which bound the state's reimbursement system together, for it represented a shared commitment to ensuring access for the uninsured and maintaining the fiscal viability of urban medical centers. From 1982 to 1988, Medicare also participated in the state's all-payer system and shouldered its share of uncompensated care. Federal officials at the Health Care Financing Administration declined to renew the Medicare waiver, leaving the other payers to pick up Medicare's share of the state's free care and bad debt pool.

By 1990 the same fears which had prompted hospitals to embrace rate regulation had resurfaced; plagued by a rising number of uninsured patients and sharp increases in bad debt, urban hospitals once again faced a fiscal crisis (Berliner and Delgado 1991). Payers were also unhappy with the system, for the state was forced to double the surcharge on hospital rates imposed on the participating third-party payers to fund the rising cost of uncompensated care. In the end, dissatisfied payers sued for relief in federal court, leading the state legislature to push through a hastily drafted reform bill fundamentally altering the state's role in health care financing (Cantor 1993). The lesson of New Jersey's experience is clear—an inequitable distribution of costs and benefits within a policy regime creates an unstable, and ultimately untenable, situation for its stakeholders. In the face of rising costs, the collective responsibility which bound providers, payers, and the state together yielded to economic self-interest, and the system collapsed.

Industry Trends

Changes in the organization and delivery of medical services may also destabilize a policy regime, for new patterns of medical practice and treatment have immediate fiscal repercussions for providers and third-party payers. For example, the shift from inpatient to outpatient hospital care over the past two decades profoundly changed the nature of hospitals' revenue stream. New inpatient treatment modalities rendered cost-control systems based on inpatient revenues (e.g., per diem rate-setting) obsolete, for a growing percentage of patients returned home after surgery that previously would have required a lengthy hospitalization. Declining length of stay also presented a major challenge for hospitals, for as less complicated (and hence more profitable) patients were treated on an outpatient basis, hospitals' inpatient population was increasingly dominated by older and sicker patients who consumed more resources.

In part, changes in the average length of stay and the growing popularity of outpatient surgery reflect the impact of managed care plans over the past decade. The expansion of managed care generated new incentives for health care providers to minimize the use of expensive specialty services, diagnostic tests, and inpatient hospital stays. In addition, since MCO contracts with providers were not included in many state rate-setting systems, managed care market penetration also limited the ability of state rate-setting programs to control systemwide costs. Managed care also reshaped the relationships among hospitals, for MCOs sought to promote price competition among providers within a region. By funneling patients (and hence revenue) to low-cost providers, MCOs threatened the fiscal health of urban medical centers and other institutions with higher than average costs. As a result, the "live and let live" spirit of collaboration which characterized many local hospital markets in the 1970s increasingly gave way to intense price-driven competition over market share.

The growth of managed care also illustrates the critical importance of providers' case mix and payer mix for the continued stability of a health care financing regime. Since the advent of prospective reimbursement using diagnosis related groups (DRGs), hospital administrators have constantly monitored the severity and complexity of cases treated by their institutions. Trauma centers and other providers that treated a disproportionate share of complicated or high-cost procedures found themselves in financial distress, for DRG-based reimbursement systems pay providers on the basis of the average cost for a procedure. Institutions which treated a higher than average number of trauma patients or AIDS cases, however, frequently found themselves with above average costs for patient care. As a result, such institutions found it increasingly difficult to compete for more profitable patients insured by private carriers and MCOs, leading to a fiscal crisis for many of the nation's trauma centers in the early 1990s.

The growth of managed care thus penalizes tertiary-care facilities and teaching institutions that offer a wide range of high-cost specialty services while rewarding low-cost "generalist" providers such as suburban community hospitals. Since teaching hospitals and tertiary-care facilities serve as the linchpin for state Emergency Medical Services (EMS) and trauma systems, the threatened closure, consolidation, or downsizing of a state's teaching hospitals can generate calls for immediate action to "bail out" financially ailing institutions. Under these circumstances, existing alliances among payers, providers, and the state may fray as policymakers explore new paths to forestall hospital closures.

The Impact of Federal Policies

Intergovernmental influences on state policy may also lead to fundamental changes in the organizing principles of a policy regime. Since state policies are formulated within the contours of a federal system, changes in federal policy often have immediate and far-reaching implications for defining the nature of policy problems at the state level. Medicaid, for example, operates as fifty separate state programs that must follow a core set of eligibility criteria, benefits, and reimbursement rules specified by federal policymakers. While it is possible for states to offer additional services beyond the mandated federal benefits package, states may not deny beneficiaries access to basic services or modify their payment methodologies without prior approval from the Health Care Financing Administration (HCFA) or Congress. Furthermore, states typically accept accreditation and quality assurance procedures specified by the federal Medicare and Medicaid programs as a means of certifying eligible providers and diagnosing fundamental problems with patient care.

Furthermore, shifts in federal policy frequently change the relative appeal of different policy instruments. Federal waiver programs and new interpretations of existing statutes can provide strong incentives for states to follow a particular path toward cost control. Prior to 1993, only Arizona had received permission to enroll all eligible Medicaid beneficiaries in managed care organizations; managed care demonstrations approved during the 1980s were limited in scope. More radical proposals, such as Oregon's plan to limit the availability of health care services to Medicaid beneficiaries as a means of expanding coverage for the uninsured, were rejected or placed in limbo during the Bush administration. Beginning in 1993, however, the Clinton administration signaled a new willingness to expand the use of its waiver authority under Section 1115 of the Social Security Act. Within two years, more than twenty states applied for Medicaid waivers to enroll eligible beneficiaries in managed care plans and/or modify the basic benefits package offered to enrollees. Federal officials, in short, sent a clear message to governors and legislators, encouraging state innovation and leading several states to embrace managed care as their principal cost-control strategy.

The Employee Retirement Income Security Act of 1974 (Pub. L. 93–406) remains one of the most significant constraints on state cost-containment efforts. The crux of the problem lies in ERISA's "preemption clause," which prohibits "any and all state laws insofar as they may now or hereafter relate to any employee benefit plan." Although the ERISA preemption clause has been criticized as "a veritable Sargasso sea of obfuscation" (Jordan 1996) the courts have interpreted the scope of its preemption mandate broadly for more than a decade. A broad interpretation of ERISA effectively precluded state efforts to expand coverage to the uninsured by requiring employers to offer health insurance to their employees (Chirba-Martin and Brennan 1994). Without an exemption, ambitious state health care reform plans in Massachusetts, Minnesota, Oregon, and Washington stalled in their tracks, for policymakers in each state supported a "pay or play" system to achieve universal health insurance coverage. Furthermore, the decisions of federal district and appeals courts in recent years threatened the legitimacy of state rate-setting programs and uncompensated care pools.[8] The U.S. Supreme Court upheld the rights of states to regulate the charges paid by insurance companies in 1995, effectively turning back a basic challenge to the ability of states to regulate the behavior of third-party health insurers.

The implication of the decision in *New York State Conference of Blue Cross and Blue Shield Plans, et al. v. Travelers Insurance Co.* suggests that the courts will uphold state laws that have only an "indirect economic effect" on employee benefit plans such as provider taxes and patient surcharges intended to reimburse hospitals for the cost of free care and bad debt attributable to uninsured patients (Jordan 1996). Since Congress has shown little inclination to limit ERISA's preemption clause through legislation, however, future challenges to state cost-containment efforts are likely. Furthermore, Congress has been unreceptive to state appeals for ad hoc exemptions from ERISA that would permit individual states to create single-payer financing systems, mandatory health insurance purchasing cooperatives that offer a standardized package of benefits, or employee mandated health insurance coverage. In short, ERISA remains a fundamental obstacle to state-level policy innovation.

Policy Images

The definition of policy problems often changes over time. Public concern about the significance of health care cost inflation and the severity and relevance of rising costs for individuals, families, and businesses leads to calls for government efforts to control health care spending. Furthermore, once the public and affected interests have acknowledged that government has a role in controlling health care costs, the prevailing problem definition will circumscribe both the means and the ends of policy (Rochefort and Cobb 1993). The shared understanding of a policy problem constitutes what Baumgartner and Jones (1991, 1993) describe as its "policy image." By defining and redefining the images of a policy or program, public officials and interest groups can shape the public's understanding of complex regulatory issues. Public perceptions of policy alternatives in either favorable or unfavorable terms (Baumgartner and Jones 1991, 1046–48) are important for building coalitions and gaining support from policymakers, for both elites and the public often seek to simplify complicated issues through the use of symbols. For example, proposals which seek to delegate authority to state agencies to regulate the rates of reimbursement for health care providers can be defined either as an effective means of controlling costs or as the latest example of "excessive" government intervention in the "free market." The fate of proposals to regulate reimbursement therefore depends on which "causal story" is accepted by decision makers, the media, and the public.

State cost-containment strategies reflect the prevailing "images" associated with the policy problem and the state's choice of policy instruments. Shifting policy images, or problem definitions, of issues define the range of acceptable policy solutions (Baumgartner and Jones 1991). Since policies are typically defined in either positive or negative terms, changes in the prevailing policy image alter both public perceptions of policy problems and expectations as to government's role in solving them. New Jersey's experience with hospital rate regulation over the past two decades illustrates the importance of policy images in establishing the terms of debates over state health care policy. In the mid-1970s, interested legislators and bureaucrats within the state's

Department of Health succeeded in defining the policy agenda in terms favorable to the expansion of public authority. In this view, ineffective regulation administered by the hospital industry had produced runaway costs; the solution, reformers argued, was a more extensive regulatory system covering all payers. Lured by the promise of federal funds for uncompensated care, state legislators, payers, and urban hospitals hailed the advent of all-payer rate-setting. A decade later, however, the system was under attack, as the solution to the policy problems of the 1970s was itself seen as the problem. A similar phenomenon occurred in Massachusetts, where soon after its passage the state's universal health care bill was vilified as a millstone around the neck of the state's economy. Universal health insurance served as a powerful rallying call for Democratic legislators and the Dukakis administration prior to the 1988 presidential election; its passage was touted as one of Michael Dukakis' principal accomplishments during his years as governor. After 1990, however, the pathbreaking legislation was increasingly viewed as a symbol of an unaffordable and unworkable policy by policymakers, providers, and the public.

PRECIPITATING FACTORS OF REGIME CHANGE

Every policy regime reflects the prevailing balance of power between the state and societal groups. Since regimes determine " who has access to political power, and how those who are in power deal with those who are not" (Fishman 1990, 428), changes in the distribution of influence within a regime can either strengthen or weaken support for state involvement in controlling health care costs. The catalysts discussed above set in motion a process of change amplified and focused by shifts in (1) the dominant political ideology among public and private decision makers; (2) partisan control of policy-making institutions; (3) coalitions of providers, payers, and other societal groups; (4) the administrative capacity of state actors; and (5) new interpretations of the state's statutory powers by federal or state courts. Shifts in one or more of these intervening variables can produce a new balance of power among payers, providers, and other non-state actors.

Political Ideology

Legislators, bureaucrats, and other state policymakers do not act in a vacuum. The range of potential policy alternatives in a state reflects the perceptions of decision makers about the limits of public authority and the proper role of government, both in terms of past practice and current opinion. A state's policy choices reflect the prevailing values and ideology shared by policymakers and the public. These values define the political culture of a state (Elazar 1974; Lowery and Sigelman 1982; Klingman and Lammers 1984), shape public perceptions of policy problems and narrow the range of acceptable policy choices to control costs. A state's political culture thus defines a set of shared values which establishes the context for policy debates.[9]

State political ideology is most likely to structure policy choices during periods of crisis, when policymakers are forced to choose among fundamentally different policy options to meet new contingencies (Higgs 1987). Prevailing beliefs about the proper role of government in the economy are reflected in informal patterns of behavior and shared understandings among members of a policy subsystem.[10] These shared understandings lead to a general predisposition for either a laissez-faire approach to policy problems or a more active government role. Even if government intervention is generally accepted as legitimate by voters and decision-making elites, ideology may shape the form of intervention (e.g., controls or incentives) used to achieve policy goals.

Support for deregulation, in particular, has a strong ideological appeal to conservative candidates and voters. In states where attitudes among voters, candidates, and other members of the health care policy-issue network shift to the right, regulatory initiatives that previously enjoyed widespread support may become politically vulnerable. Ideology is most likely to reshape the policy-making environment in states where the views of academic experts, policymakers, and the public converge. Under these circumstances, "the politics of ideas" (Derthick and Quirk 1985) can lead to calls for a fundamental shift in government policy toward the health care industry. When consensus among experts and industry groups is lacking, however, the power of ideology to redefine relationships between state and society is more limited, for both supporters and opponents are able to marshal "experts" to defend their definition of the policy problem.

Furthermore, ideology is most likely to play a significant role in uprooting established patterns of regulatory politics when used by political candidates or policymakers as a framework to set the agenda for a campaign, legislative session, or term. Candidates who define issues in ideological terms are able upon entering office to claim a popular mandate for their agenda that may be used to build legislative support for changing established policies. The power of ideology to set the legislative agenda became readily apparent in the early 1990s as newly elected conservative Republican governors moved quickly to "downsize" government in many states. In Massachusetts, for example, Governor William Weld halted implementation of the universal health care law passed by his predecessor, Michael Dukakis, and won passage of legislation to deregulate the state's hospital industry. Elsewhere in the region, both New Jersey Governor Christine Whitman and New York Governor George Pataki attacked government regulatory programs as inefficient; both promoted competition and a smaller, leaner government as the solution to rising health care costs in tight fiscal times.

Partisan Shifts

The role of political parties in shaping state policy choices remains a matter of intense debate. In part, the continued controversy over the impact of party on policy is based on the expectation that Democratic control of state government institutions is associated with more liberal state policies than Republican control. However, since the ideological positions of Democratic and Republican parties differ from state to state, partisanship is likely to be a poor predictor of policy liberalism (Erikson, Wright, and McIver 1989). The ability of legislative parties to counterbalance the influence of organized interests is limited. While legislators possess considerable discretion in making policy, party leaders are inclined to agree with group positions when they become involved in conflicts over issues (Wiggins, Hamm, and Bell 1992). In addition, the influence of party leaders is subject to change, and the relative importance of the governor and majority legislative leadership varies over time (Wiggins, Hamm, and Bell 1992).

Numerous studies of social welfare policy over the past three decades (see Plotnick and Winters 1985; Dye 1984) also suggest that neither party control nor interparty competition has a strong impact on state policy. Partisanship becomes relevant, however, when candidates or legislative leaders stake out distinctive issue positions. Policy liberalism, therefore, depends on the presence of "policy relevant parties" (Dye 1984). Unless parties are ideologically differentiated, variations in party control are unlikely to produce dramatic policy change. Partisan realignments, however, can unseat entrenched supporters of a regime, leading to sudden shifts in the policy-making environment. The impact of partisan change is particularly clear in New York, where the election of George Pataki in 1994 led to dramatic policy reversals in education funding, taxes, intergovernmental aid, and health care financing.

Issue Networks

The complexity and technical detail which accompanies most discussions of hospital rate-setting and certificate-of-need regulation resembles Gormley's (1986) description of "boardroom politics" in which decision-making rests in the hands of bureaucrats, professionals, and business groups. Indeed, the decision-making process for most health policy issues has been described as an "unbalanced political market" biased in favor of health care providers and payers (Marmor, Heagy, and Litman 1976). Unbalanced political markets emerge in many regulatory arenas because groups with a "concentrated" interest in an issue have a greater incentive to engage in political activity than those who have a smaller stake in the outcome (Wilson 1973, 1980). While public interest groups played a prominent role in policy formulation during the debate over Massachusetts' universal health care legislation in the late 1980s, they have been notably absent elsewhere (Goldberger 1990).

One of the most significant changes in state health policy-making over the past decade has been the growing role of business groups in health policy debates. In recent years, corporate leaders (Bergthold 1990a) and business-led health care coalitions (McLaughlin, Zellers, and Brown 1989) have been in the vanguard of reform, and business-sponsored think tanks and peak associations have become active participants in debates over insurance reforms, managed care, rate-setting, and capital expenditure review. The political activism of business has followed two principal paths as corporations and peak associations engaged in legislative lobbying and in efforts to augment their purchasing power in private markets. In Massachusetts, the business community followed the former strategy, as prominent CEOs brokered a compromise among providers, payers, and state officials which led to the creation of the state's all-payer rate-setting system in 1982 (Bergthold 1988). Elsewhere, however, businesses have embraced private rather than public solutions to control their health care costs. In Tennessee, for example, local employers invited hospitals to bid for contracts to provide hospital care for more than 25,000 employees and developed an exclusive contract with the successful bidder (Winslow 1992). In other states, business coalitions have created purchasing alliances, published data on hospital costs and utilization for members, or turned to self-insurance as a means of controlling the rising cost of employee fringe benefits. If businesses are unable to control costs through private initiatives, they will turn to public officials for assistance. Since some policy-making environments are more responsive to public solutions than others, business will be more involved in the legislative process in states with more extensive government intervention in health care financing.

Changes in the formal representation and participation of interest groups may also contribute to the transformation of a policy regime. Decisions about representation on reform commissions and advisory commissions often have long-lasting consequences, for these institutions often define the policy problems and establish legislative priorities for elected officials and relevant publics. The importance of diversity in policy-making reflects Schattschneider's (1960, 20) observation that "nearly all theories about politics have something to do with the question of who can get into the fight and who is to be excluded." If agenda-setting or policy-making bodies are dominated by one group or collection of groups, public officials will be more likely to represent the views expressed by the well organized at the expense of others who are not well represented in policy debates (see McConnell 1966; Lowi 1969; Wilson 1980).

Health care policy-making reflects the diversity and density of a state's interest group system (Gray and Lowery 1993a, 1993b). The permeability of policy regimes may be assessed by determining if all groups which may be significantly affected by a proposed policy are included within the state's health care policy-issue network (Berry 1994). The entry of business, or any new groups, into state health policy debates has the potential to destabilize established relationships among public and private actors in a policy regime. By aligning with third-party payers and the state, businesses can bolster nascent efforts to control costs by facilitating the development of a public-private partnership for reform. In other states, however, business leaders have led the fight against regulation of health care providers or emerged as key proponents of deregulation. In short, changes in the composition of interest groups within a policy regime can lead to the formation of new political alliances and the disruption of existing ones.

Issue networks at the state level can be dominated either by state officials or by private advocacy coalitions, which may be either cohesive or fragmented. When state officials and private interests have strongly held policy preferences, the outcome of these conflicts will be shaped by the ability of public and private actors to mobilize support for their preferred policies (see Cobb and Elder 1982). The ability of state officials to resist societal pressures or overcome concerted opposition from relevant publics is contingent upon the cohesiveness of industry advocacy coalitions. Where the hospital industry is highly cohesive and businesses and other nonproviders remain fragmented, providers will retain the upper hand in policy debates. Under these circumstances, hospitals often seek to limit competition by opposing the entry of new providers and to resist attempts to impose rate regulation, capitation, or other limits on hospital revenues (Imershein, Rond, and Mathis 1992, 976–77). In contrast, where sharp divisions exist among health care elites, other parties have an opportunity either to impose regulation upon the industry to control costs or to negotiate discounts on prices (Imershein, Rond, and Mathis 1992, 978).

Where issue networks include two or more competing advocacy

coalitions, policy development and implementation will be shaped by the relative influence of the participating groups (May 1991). Fissures within existing political coalitions can also undermine support for a regime, as changes in state policy or private bargaining often pit former allies against each other by creating zero sum conflicts over reimbursement. In New Jersey, for example, the deteriorating fiscal health of urban medical centers led many teaching hospitals to embrace an all-payer rate-setting system in the 1970s as a means of financing the spiraling cost of uncompensated care (Morone and Dunham 1985). While the industry had vehemently opposed state regulation of hospital rates in the late 1960s and early 1970s, by the end of the decade urban and suburban hospitals parted company; by pitting the interests of affluent community hospitals against the pressing fiscal needs of urban teaching institutions, the proposed DRG reimbursement system opened the door to state regulation on an unprecedented scale.

The Administrative Capacity of the State

Over time, changes in the professional expertise of public officials, the stability of policy-making institutions, and the specialization of state policy-making institutions can shift the balance of power in a policy regime. State administrative capacities are not static, but expand and contract over time with changes in funding, personnel policies, and policy priorities. In many states, capacity-building grants from the federal government or private foundations provided the impetus for hiring of talented professionals to develop new programs or expand existing ones. Such efforts are doomed to fail, however, if states decline to incorporate funding for these positions into the budget once outside funding sources have dried up. Insufficient staff, budget cutbacks, or low salaries relative to the private sector hinder the ability of state governments to attract and retain key personnel. Under these circumstances, state agencies are likely to become a "training ground" for the private sector, for the most talented or experienced individuals will find it difficult to resist the lure of better salaries and support offered by providers, third-party payers, or private lobbying groups. A high rate of personnel turnover in state agencies also limits the ability of public officials to counteract the private sector's advantages in information and expertise. Over time, high turnover will erode the ability of states to undertake major policy initiatives or implement existing tasks (Sapolsky, Aisenberg, and Morone 1987). When the state's resources are overwhelmed by the private sector, the stage is set for interest groups to dominate the policy-making process.

Frequent changes in leadership can create uncertainty among client groups over the agency's direction and policy priorities. Leadership stability is also vital for the ongoing success of state regulation, for "without creative political leadership, new strategic opportunities for action do not bear fruit" (Skowronek 1982, 171). Effective leaders can energize an organization by clearly defining a unifying sense of purpose and mission or by mobilizing support for their goals among significant external constituencies (Doig and Hargrove 1987). This leadership can take many forms, from charismatic public salesmanship to behind-the-scenes efforts at coalition-building, but in either case, stability in top management positions greatly enhances an organization's credibility.

Conversely, the departure of key figures from the state health care policy-issue network can fundamentally alter the dynamics of policy-making in a state, particularly if the departing individuals played a vital role in defining policy choices or mediating group conflicts. In New Jersey, the departure of Health Commissioner Joann Finley and the other principal architects of the state's DRG-based payment methodology sharply limited the ability of the Department of Health to refine its all-payer rate-setting system (Sapolsky, Aisenberg, and Morone 1987). Similarly, the unexpected resignation of Commissioner David Axelrod after a stroke in 1991 created a massive void in New York's health policy regime; for more than a decade, Axelrod had redefined the health policy agenda in the Empire State to focus on cost containment and quality assurance. In the six years since Axelrod's resignation, health care policy-making in New York has undergone a wrenching transformation as the Department of Health lost much of its former influence over the policy process. As Bruce Vladeck, the president of the United Hospital Fund, observed in 1991, the commissioner "so dominated issues of health policy in this state for the last decade that there's a real sense of drift and uncertainty and anxiety about where we're going on these important issues" (quoted in Sack 1991, B1).

The Courts

Without a basic consensus over the proper scope of government authority, the implementation and administration of payment rates and regulations will be characterized by an endless series of lawsuits and appeals with aggrieved parties lining up to challenge the "rules of the game" in court. The decisions of state or federal courts, in turn, delineate the legitimate scope of state authority. Judges have played a vital role in circumscribing the exercise of state power from the nineteenth century's "state of courts and parties" (Skowronek 1982) to the present. Contemporary state and federal courts continue to redefine the relationship between state and market in the health sector, as evident in recent court decisions invalidating state assessments on health care providers to fund uncompensated care for the uninsured in New York, New Jersey, and Connecticut.[11] On the other hand, some courts have upheld the powers of states to set rates of reimbursement, approve the introduction of new technologies, or to decrease the number of hospital beds to conform with state health planning objectives.[12]

Prior to 1992, New Jersey's health care financing system reflected a commitment to controlling health care costs through state rate regulation, subsidizing care for the uninsured and indigent, and supporting distressed urban teaching hospitals (Cantor 1993). Labor unions challenged the legality of the state's system of financing uncompensated care, arguing that the state surcharge on inpatient hospital bills violated the provisions of the Employee Income and Retirement Security Act of 1974 (ERISA). While the U.S. Supreme Court later upheld the right of states to impose surcharges on all payers for public purposes, the decision by the lower court prompted state legislators to undertake a sweeping revision of the state's hospital payment system. The end result was a fundamental restructuring of the state's policy regime; the principles which had shaped policy-making for more than a decade were cast aside. Within six months of the Court's decision, the New Jersey legislature enacted a sweeping reform package which deregulated hospital rates, reduced state subsidies for indigent care, and distributed the state's uncompensated care fund (which had previously given preference to distressed hospitals) among the state's community and teaching hospitals (Cantor 1993). In short, the goals and principles which led to the creation of the state's all-payer system in the late 1970s were abandoned in favor of a market-oriented approach to controlling costs and a limited system of insurance subsidies for the working poor.

The judiciary has also shaped state policy on the level of payments to providers. In 1986, hospitals in Virginia challenged the validity of the state's Medicaid reimbursement rates, which they contended were not "reasonable and adequate" as required by the Boren Amendment to the Medicaid program. The Court's decision in *Wilder v. Virginia* in 1990 limited the ability of states to impose restrictive payment schedules on health care providers; in the majority opinion, Justice Brennan argued that the Boren Amendment entitled hospitals to be paid "reasonable and adequate rates to meet the cost of an efficient and economical health care provider." While the Court left decisions about the reasonableness and adequacy of rates, and criteria for assessing the efficiency of health care providers, to the states, it affirmed the right of providers to sue public officials for relief. Nevertheless, the scope of state powers to regulate health care financing or the contracting practices of HMOs and other providers remains vulnerable to legal challenges at both the state and federal level.

CHANGE AND CONTINUITY IN THE
NORTHEASTERN STATES

The changing politics of state efforts to control health care costs are best illustrated by a comparative case study methodology. The following chapters explore the evolution of health policy regimes in Massachusetts, New Hampshire, New York, and Rhode Island over the past two decades. The case study chapters present an overview of each state's health care financing system and describe the essential characteristics of the policy-making process using the regime framework described in Chapter 1. In addition, each chapter seeks to account for changes over time in state cost-containment strategies and in the larger relationship between state officials and societal groups. Internal contradictions challenged the stability of each state's policy regime on at least one occasion over the past decade, but while regimes in Massachusetts and New York weakened considerably in recent years, those in New Hampshire and Rhode Island have been characterized by stability and mutual adjustment among public and private interests within their respective issue networks. Since the four states under study represent all three regime types discussed in Chapter 1, the Northeastern states offer an unusual opportunity to study the dynamics of regime change.

All four states have experienced conflict over technical or procedural issues. While conflict within regimes is to be expected among players in a multibillion-dollar industry, in two states—Massachusetts and New York—disagreements over the administration of state policies led to fundamental challenges to the norms and principles which governed the regime. In contrast, regimes in New Hampshire and Rhode Island emerged unscathed from changes in federal policies and industry trends over the past two decades, as public and private actors continued to support the underlying principles and norms of each state's health policy regime. The continuity of the policy-making process in both states, as well as the dramatic changes in policy which occurred in Massachusetts and New York, illustrate the model of policy change described above.

Since 1990, health care policy-making in Massachusetts and New York has undergone a series of wrenching changes. These developments raise a variety of questions about how and why regimes change. Republican victories in gubernatorial races precipitated radical policy changes in Massachusetts and New York, but had little impact in Rhode Island. Similarly, while state hospital rate-setting programs lost legitimacy in the eyes of key societal groups during the late 1980s in Massachusetts and New York, the policy image of Rhode Island's unique rate-setting methodology continued to win the support of public and private groups. The importance of power shifts within policy regimes is also evident in a comparative study of the Northeastern states, for health care policy issue networks in Massachusetts and New York have been much more permeable than those in New Hampshire and Rhode Island. For example, business groups emerged as a potent political force on health care financing issues in Massachusetts and New York but remained on the sidelines in New Hampshire and Rhode Island during the 1980s. Despite their differences, however, all four Northeastern states have successfully applied for Medicaid waivers under Section 1115 since 1993.

Chapter 3 explores the politics of the reimbursement process in New York, where soaring expenses for Medicaid and chronic health care inflation led to the development of an imposed regime during the 1970s. Over the past two decades, hospitals in New York have operated within one of the most intensely regulated health care financing systems in the nation. With strong support for regulatory controls from the executive branch, the legislature, and the courts, public officials in the New York Department of Health created one of the most stringent payment systems in the United States to control costs and increase access to care for the uninsured. For more than two decades, public officials possessed a well-defined commitment to controlling costs which was developed and implemented despite vehement protests from health care providers. By the early 1990s, however, New York's health policy regime was weakened by a confluence of internal and external challenges. By 1995, support for the state's imposed regulatory regime collapsed, paving the way for the deregulation of the state's payment system and a fundamental shift in the relationship between state officials and societal groups.

Massachusetts' experience illustrates the dilemmas of policy-making under a negotiated regime. Chapter 4 examines both the meso-corporatist origins of the state's negotiated regime in the early 1980s and its subsequent implosion later in the decade. The deregulation of the state's payment system in the early 1990s, however, left many vestiges of the state's universal health insurance act in place. Changes in Massachusetts' health policy regime illustrate the importance of state administrative capacities and the permeability of state issue networks as agents of policy change. Fiscal crisis and an ideological shift within the executive branch emerged as pivotal factors in explaining policy change within the Bay State's negotiated regime since 1990. Despite fundamental changes in its cost-containment strategy, health care policy-making in Massachusetts continues to be governed by a negotiated regime. While the form of state intervention has changed over time, state officials have not yet abrogated policy-making responsibilities to the marketplace.

Chapter 5 offers an opportunity to explore the roots of policy stability within the contours of a negotiated regime. In Rhode Island, the ability of public officials to change provider behavior is limited by both institutional and ideological constraints. Although different in form from its northern neighbor, health care regulation in Rhode Island is also governed by a negotiated regime; with few participants and a (relatively) congenial relationship among affected interest groups and state government, policy-making has a strong corporatist flavor. Underlying tensions, however, undermined the ability of the state to effectively control costs through its unique approach to rate setting, and ultimately derailed its aggressive regulation of providers' capital investments. Nevertheless, the state's unique reimbursement system has operated successfully for more than two decades without significant challenges to its legitimacy. Conflicts over health care policy have revolved around technical or procedural issues; none of the principal public or private actors in the state's health care policy-issue network has contested the basic norms or principles of the regime.

In Chapter 6, health care policy-making in New Hampshire offers a contemporary example of a market regime. The relationship between providers, payers, and the state is fundamentally different under a market regime, where public officials possess little formal authority to regulate the hospital industry. Under these circumstances, state government is poorly positioned to be a catalyst of change, for in the spirit of Grant McConnell's (1966) "orthodox tradition," the prevailing political culture favors private solutions to public problems as both more efficient and less threatening than state intervention. Consensus on ideological and programmatic goals among participants and relevant publics in the health care policy-issue network remains high, for the state imposes few requirements on either providers or payers; responsibility for negotiating reimbursement rates rests squarely with the private sector.

CHAPTER NOTES

1. Goldberger (1990) offers a different view of the importance of citizens groups in Massachusetts during the debate over the Health Security Act in 1987–88.

2. For a dissenting view, see Almond (1988) and Ellis (1992).

3. Despite protests that pluralists did not deny the importance of public officials (Almond 1988; Ellis 1992), the principal shortcoming of pluralist models is one of emphasis. The preferences of public officials and the structure of political institutions are not accorded much weight in explaining policy outcomes in most pluralist accounts.

4. In Offe's (1981) view, political systems can be defined as more or less corporatist, "depending on the extent to which public status is attributed to private interest groups." The attribution of public status to interest groups, in turn, depends upon the degree to which the resources of constituent organizations are supported by the state, the regulation of organizational operating charters and internal organization, and the extent to which groups are licensed or formally recognized by the state as participants in the development, implementation, or administration of policy (Offe 1981, 136–37).

5. Schmitter (1979, 13) defines corporatism as a "system of interest intermediation in which the constituent groups are organized into a limited number of singular, compulsory, noncompetitive, hierarchically ordered, and functionally differentiated categories, recognized or licensed (if not created) by the state, and granted a deliberate representational monopoly within their respective categories in exchange for observing certain controls on their selection of leaders and articulation of demands and supports."

6. Several factors limited the impact of competition on hospital prices. First, since HMO market share ("penetration") in most states remained well below 20% during the 1980s, managed care arrangements did not force providers to significantly alter their behavior. Even in markets with high rates of HMO membership, managed care plans tended to "shadow price" traditional indemnity products (Luft, Maerki, and Trauner 1986). Finally, consumers' willingness to shift health insurers to take advantage of price differentials is limited; fewer than 10% of elderly Medicare beneficiaries opted to switch plans despite the promise of considerable cost savings (Kronick 1992).

7. Young (1983, 107) defines regime transformation as "significant alterations in a regime's structure of rights and rules, the character of its social choice mechanisms, and the nature of its compliance mechanisms."

8. See the courts' decisions in *Travelers' Insurance Co. v. Cuomo*, 14 F.3d 708 (2nd Circuit, 1993); *Travelers Insurance Co. v. Cuomo*, 813 F. Supp. 996 (S.D.N.Y. 1993). An earlier decision by the Court of Appeals (2nd Circuit) in the case of *Rebaldo v. Cuomo*, 749 F.2d 133 (2nd circuit, 1984), upheld New York's hospital rate-setting system and effectively quashed the efforts of dissatisfied providers and payers to challenge the constitutionality of the state's reimbursment system. In its decision in *Travelers*, however, the Court of Appeals held that "Rebaldo's entire analysis is poisoned by its discredited belief that ERISA's preemption clause is targeted only at state laws that 'purport to regulate' plan terms and conditions." This interpretation, if affirmed by the U.S. Supreme Court, would have effectively invalidated the Empire State's entire rate-setting methodology.

9. Jacobs (1992, 186) argues that "culture is a mediating factor, or 'middle-term' between environmental conditions (such as administrative capacity and economic or class forces) and human behavior. Culture represents the subjective orientations by which members of a society can understand and respond to their environment."

10. A state's political ideology can be defined as the aggregate issue preferences of the population placed on a liberal/conservative continuum (Holbrook-Provow and Poe 1987). Similarly, state predispositions for enacting innovative

or progressive policies in a variety of issue areas, which Klingman and Lammers (1984) describe as "general policy liberalism," offer a summary indicator of government activism. Steven Rosenstone's noted that a state's commitment to "New Deal social welfare liberalism" in providing social services also serves as an indicator of policy liberalism or conservatism (Holbrook-Provow and Poe 1987, 405). Both general policy liberalism and Rosenstone's measure of the generosity of state social welfare programs, however, suggest that a liberal orientation toward social problems in one issue area may "spill over" into other policy domains.

11. See the decision by the U.S. Court of Appeals (3rd Circuit) in *United Wire, Metal and Machine Health and Welfare Fund v. Morristown Memorial Hospital*, 995 F.2d 1179 (3d Cir. 1993) and the U.S. Supreme Court's majority opinion in *New York State Conference of Blue Cross and Blue Shield Plans, et al. v. Travelers Insurance Co.*, 115 S.Ct. 1671 (1995).

12. See *Rebaldo v. Cuomo*, 749 F.2d 133 (2nd circuit, 1984) with respect to rate-setting and Roos' (1987) excellent analysis of challenges to state certificate-of-need laws.

3

New York:
The Transformation of an
Imposed Policy Regime

For more than thirty years, state officials in New York pursued authoritative solutions to control health care costs that sharply curtailed the autonomy of health care providers and third-party payers. Until the deregulation of hospital rates in 1996, the fiscal health of providers in New York was determined by highly contentious legislative negotiations over reimbursement. Under these circumstances, the managerial autonomy of hospital administrators was severely limited. New York's imposed regulatory regime has its roots in the state's recurring fiscal crises over the past two decades. Although the state's "top-down" decision-making process was widely criticized by the hospital industry, New York's stringent rate-setting methodology and capital expenditure controls enjoyed strong support from both the governor's office and the legislature. Furthermore, the professionalization of the state's health care bureaucracy and legislature enabled New York to refine and adapt its payment system over time in response to changes in its environment.

New York's long history of regulatory activism in health care dates back to its early health planning efforts in the mid-1960s. The passage of the Metcalf-McClosky Act (Chapter 730 of the New York Public Laws of 1964) required hospitals and other health providers to obtain approval from the state's Department of Social Welfare for the construction of new capital projects and for changes in services or numbers of beds. Within two decades, New York's hospital industry became one of the most heavily regulated in the nation, and the state served as the model for the federal Health Planning and Resource Development Act (Pub. L. 93-641). State regulation of Blue Cross and Medicaid rates began with the passage of New York's first rate-setting program (Chapter 957 of the New York Public Laws of 1969), which used peer-group comparisons among similar institutions to determine reimbursement rates for inpatient care. This legislation established a precedent, continued to the present day, which encourages the efficient production of hospital services.

Fiscal crises during the 1970s prompted New York to impose increasingly stringent cost ceilings on reimbursement rates. This culminated in a freeze on outpatient Medicaid reimbursement (Chapter 76 of the New York Public Laws of 1976) and the Charge Control Act of 1978, which limited annual increases in hospital charges to a fixed percentage, or trend factor. In 1982, the Empire State received a waiver authorizing Medicare's participation in an all-payer, per diem rate-setting system from the Health Care Financing Administration. After the expiration of the Medicare waiver three years later, New York continued to operate its per diem system for all other payers until the state moved to a new case-based reimbursement system using diagnosis-related groups in 1988.

By the mid-1990s, however, health care policy-making in New York was in a state of flux. The election of a conservative Republican governor, George Pataki, and significant changes in the organization and delivery of health care in New York contributed to public and private calls for reforming the state's complex health care financing system. The Pataki administration has emphasized managed care, rather than rate-setting and other regulatory controls, as the most effective means of controlling the state's massive Medicaid budget. In particular, the state has submitted a Medicaid managed care waiver application to enroll the vast majority of its caseload in capitated plans in an effort to harness market forces to control program costs. The most sweeping change in state policy, however, occured in 1996, when legislators endorsed a comprehensive proposal to deregulate hospital payment rates as of January 1, 1997. Health care policy-making in New York is now in transition, for while the state continues to be actively involved in funding medical education, uncompensated care, and subsidized insurance for low-income residents, policymakers have abandoned regulatory controls in favor of market competition as the principal means of controlling health care costs.

THE POLICY-MAKING ENVIRONMENT IN NEW YORK STATE

Hospitals in New York State operated within one of the nation's most heavily regulated payment systems over the past three decades. State control over hospital reimbursement has led to chronic fiscal instability within the state's hospital industry; despite rising demand for hospital services, more than 40 institutions closed their doors in the decade following New York's fiscal crisis in 1975. Over the past decade, hospitals in New York were severely limited in their ability to shift costs from one class of payers to another. Under these circumstances, industry officials lobbied heavily for the infusion of more state resources, particularly in the form of more generous reimbursement under the state's prospective-payment system. Though ailing financially, the state's hospital industry has considerable political influence as an employer of more than 330,000 New Yorkers and generates more than $25 billion in annual revenues. In particular, the Healthcare Association of New York State (HANYS) wields considerable influence in the Republican-dominated Senate. HANYS actively lobbies the legislature on all issues related to health care financing and the delivery of health services and regularly mounts grass-roots campaigns to mobilize local hospitals to pressure legislators to support the industry's positions.

In the early 1990s, these efforts paid off handsomely; extensive lobbying by HANYS and regional hospital associations enabled hospitals to add more than $300 million in additional funds to the 1990 reimbursement bill that reauthorized the state's prospective reimbursement system until 1993. Hospitals won another victory in December 1993 when the industry was able to persuade the legislature to add an additional $181 million over the amount proposed by Governor Mario Cuomo and Health Commissioner Marc Chassin during the renegotiation of the New York Prospective Hospital Reimbursement Methodology in 1993 (NYPHRM V). In the words of one senior Department of Health (DOH) official,

> the hospitals have had much more receptivity in the legislature over the past few years than they've had here in the Department. They are the second largest political action committee in the state [and] they see the legislature as their ally against the Department.

During the renegotiation of the hospital payment system in 1990, one staff member for the Business Council of New York State observed that "a lot of what happened and didn't happen was due to the strength of the hospital association." Despite Governor Cuomo's rhetoric about cost containment, he signed a HANYS-sponsored bill pumping more than $300 million of additional funding into the state's hospital industry while a more aggressive cost-containment package supported by Commissioner Axelrod and the Business Council failed to win legislative support. Political realities intervened on HANYS' behalf in 1990, however, as the governor was campaigning for reelection while the bill was under consideration. The influence of the hospital industry—and in particular, of hospital unions—over the reauthorization of the state's payment system in 1990 supports Ciangrelli's (1993, 271) observation that while business groups were often perceived as the most influential lobbying groups during "routine" legislative sessions, the unions' ability to deliver campaign workers, votes, and financial support greatly enhanced their effectiveness in election years. As one Business Council staffer noted,

> This time the legislature did the same thing that they did the last time [in 1987], but they did it when the Governor had to go to New York City to campaign for reelection and had to go to the Bronx and ask people to vote for him. They had timing on their side this year.

While HANYS emerges as the dominant legislative spokesman for the industry, the state's seven regional hospital associations are also actively involved in payment matters. The regional associations, however, tend to adopt a more parochial view, focusing their attention on the impact of state policy on their members; most prefer to concentrate their resources on local matters, leaving HANYS to articulate statewide goals and programmatic objectives for the industry as a whole.

Aside from HANYS, Empire Blue Cross and Blue Shield is the single most influential private participant in the hospital regulatory process in New York State. While there are five other Blue Cross plans in the state, Empire is more than ten times larger than its nearest competitor, Rochester Hospital Service Corp., in terms of total claims processed. The company's size makes it the de facto spokesman for the state's health insurance industry. Since more than 80% of the private insurance market in New York was controlled by the seven regional Blue Cross plans during the 1970s and 1980s, commercial insurers and HMOs were not a major political force in reimbursement debates until recent years.

Concerns about the frail fiscal position of Empire Blue Cross and Blue Shield have figured prominently in legislative debates in recent years. During 1993, the company lost more than 500,000 subscribers in the wake of a torrent of adverse publicity and continued double-digit rate increases; it saw a reduction of more than 10% of its community-rated small group members (Gottlieb 1993). In addition, Empire's initial venture into managed care through its Healthnet HMO was plagued by embarrassing administrative problems and persistent financial losses; since its introduction in the late 1980s, Healthnet was scored by both patients and providers for tardy bill processing, shortages of primary-care physicians in several counties, and an inability to establish and enforce practice standards for participating providers (Meier 1993). Despite a strong showing in fiscal year 1990, in which the plan enjoyed a surplus of $295 million, Empire Blue Cross still fell short of a critical capital test in the insurance industry since it had less than four weeks of claims coverage in surplus at year's end (Pulliam, 1991:A6). Using data obtained from Weiss Research (the only insurance rating agency which evaluates Blue Cross plans) and the national Blue Cross and Blue Shield Association, the General Accounting Office concluded in 1994 that although Empire Blue Cross and Blue Shield was no longer in "immediate danger of insolvency," it remained one of the two weakest plans in the nation (GAO 1994).

Despite its fiscal problems, the company has a strong presence in the legislature, where it employs the services of the prestigious Albany law firm of Hinsman, Straub, Pigors and Manning to promote its agenda. The company's intensive lobbying activities were particularly apparent in the debate over the 1990 reimbursement bill. In the thick of the negotiations in July, Empire Blue Cross ran full-page ads in the national edition of the *Wall Street Journal* opposing the measure. Much of the Blue Cross concern in 1990 centered on the relatively technical aspect of funding outpatient services. Under NYPHRM III, if the legislature authorized higher rates for inpatient services, Blue Cross rates would also rise. On the outpatient side, however, the rates were not linked, thereby giving Blue Cross plans the freedom to negotiate rates with providers as they saw fit. In the opinion of one hospital representative, "the Blues have not been active in policy development but really just in how things affect them. All they cared about was whether they [Medicaid and Blue Cross outpatient rates] were going to be linked or not."

The state's business community became an increasingly active participant in legislative battles during the 1980s. The principal voice of the business community in New York is the Business Council of New York State, an employer-sponsored organization and think tank based in Albany, which engages in both governmental lobbying and in the development of new programs. While the Business Council is most concerned with issues that affect the state's large corporations that underwrite its activities, its aggressive pursuit of health care cost-containment initiatives benefits both large and small firms. This is fortunate for small businesses, for the primary voice of small business, the Chamber of Commerce, has not assumed an active role in hospital regulation.

In 1988, the Business Council increased its stature as a major player in legislative politics when it was credited for persuading Governor Cuomo to veto NYPHRM III on the grounds that it was inflationary. Business Council staffers note that the governor's action enhanced their reputation and perceived influence on hospital payment issues because the council was seen as the only major organization opposing the legislation. The council's overall record is mixed, though, for while the business community contributed to the defeat of the hospital industry's pleas for more funds in 1988, business lost in 1990 when the hospitals were able to add millions of dollars to the renewal of the case-based payment system over the opposition of Health Department officials, Blue Cross, and the Business Council.

Business leaders were upset that the movement toward regional pricing that began in 1987 did not continue under NYPHRM IV. Under regional pricing, a hospital's revenue for treating a patient is based on the average cost for similar procedures, known as the group price or pricing component, at other hospitals in the region.[1] The Department of Health, supported by the state's insurance industry and other businesses, proposed to continue this trend until all hospitals were paid on the basis of a group price. The council, however, was unable to convince the legislature to continue the movement toward regional pricing during the renegotiation of the payment system in 1990. As one Business Council staffer complained, "We felt that in return for the up-front money, there should be some tit for tat. We weren't displeased with how they allocated the money (65% went into labor costs) but we were displeased with the size of the allocation in 1990."

Before 1985, the business community in New York played what officials described as a "catch-up role" in health care debates. Rising costs, however, provided the impetus for a more active role in formulating the state's health policy. In the words of one Business Council policy analyst, "When we took a look at it, it became obvious to us that the cost of hospital care on the inpatient side was such a huge component of total overall costs that it would be a good place to start." In 1987, the council's recommendations for reforming the state's payment system stated that "the issue of health care costs has consistently been identified in our surveys, along with taxes, as the key areas of concern to both the large and small business communities across the state" (Business Council 1987, 1). The legislative debate over the adoption of a case-based payment system in 1987–88 provided a foundation for the Business Council's involvement in later years and also set a particularly effective pattern in terms of legislative lobbying.

Business strategy proceeded on two levels. At the grass-roots level, the Business Council engaged in a personalized lobbying campaign with legislators and their staffs in which prominent executives contacted their local representatives and senators to "explain" the impact of exploding hospital costs on the cost of doing business in New York. As one staffer quipped, "These people aren't junior vice presidents for marketing—they're senior executives in Fortune 500 companies." At the same time, the council focused its resources on the legislature in Albany. In the words of one lobbyist for the council,

> We developed a position paper and mailed that to the full legislature, the Department of Health, and all the key decision-makers and followed that up with numerous personal visits. We spent the better part of the legislative

session in 1987 giving examples to members of how health costs were going up and outlining different approaches that we thought should be taken to minimize cost increases.

The Business Council strongly endorsed the Pataki administration's proposal to deregulate hospital costs in 1996. In a 1996 briefing paper, the council urged members to support its efforts to "move the state's antiquated system of hospital rate-setting into the open market where greater cost controls can be achieved without sacrificing quality of care for New York's residents" (Business Council 1996b). The council lobbied heavily for deregulation during the initial deliberations over reforming the health care financing system in 1995. One of the Business Council's leading spokesmen, the director of benefits for Eastman Kodak, served as a representative on Governor Pataki's Ad Hoc Task Force on NYPHRM in 1995. In addition, the council's efforts to mobilize the business community led representatives from many of the state's largest firms such as General Electric and NYNEX to testify in favor of deregulation in hearings held by the task force during 1995. As legislative debate over deregulation began in 1996, the council urged the governor and legislators to reject proposals to extend NYPHRM (Business Council 1996a).

While business interests have repeatedly been identified as one of the most powerful lobbies in New York State, "the poor, the consumers, the nonunionized workers, and the young have little voice among the lobby groups in Albany" (Ciangrelli 1993, 269). While New York has a strong and diverse interest group system (Smith 1984; Ciangrelli 1993), public interest groups and advocates for the poor have been conspicuously absent in legislative debates over reauthorizing the state's health care financing system in the past decade. As a result, the health care policy-issue network in New York resembles Gormley's (1986) description of "board-room politics," as providers, payers, and other corporate elites seek to shape the content of highly technical negotiations over reimbursement, contracting, and labor costs.

NEW YORK STATE'S APPROACH TO HOSPITAL COST CONTAINMENT

New York's first efforts to control rising health care costs sought to rationalize the delivery of hospital services through comprehensive health planning. Voluntary health planning sponsored by health insurers, hospitals, and private foundations (e.g., the United Hospital Fund) first appeared in the late 1930s. Privately sponsored planning initiatives, however, had little success in reorganizing the delivery of health service in New York, for third-party payers continued to reimburse providers using a retrospective, cost-based methodology (Fox 1991). Beginning in the late 1950s, rapid inflation in Blue Cross premiums led to the formation of a state commission to investigate the company's reimbursement procedures amid corresponding calls for action from subscribers, businesses, and legislators to slow the growth in premiums (Marmor 1991). The commission, chaired by Columbia University professor Raymond Trussell, recommended that the state license hospital construction and renovation through a formal regional planning process (Fox 1991).

Support from Blue Cross was instrumental in establishing the state's health planning system. By the late 1950s, the Associated Hospital Service (the precursor of Empire Blue Cross) was caught in a bind; as its cost-based system of reimbursement led to rapid growth in payments to providers, the state insurance department refused to grant the company's request for high premium increases (Marmor 1991, 774–75). Under these circumstances, Blue Cross opted to support a public solution to its problem and energetically pressed for state action to review the construction of new facilities and the addition of new services in the hope of restricting access to high-cost services (Marmor 1991, 777). New York became the first state in the nation to adopt certificate-of-need regulation with the passage of the Metcalf-McClosky Act (Chapter 730 of the New York Public Laws of 1964). Later in the decade, Blue Cross was also "in the forefront of those actively seeking the [introduction of] rate-setting legislation, while the hospital associations accepted the legislation as less onerous than a freezing of Medicaid rates" (Marmor 1991, 784).

The certificate-of-need (CON) review process in New York evaluates applications in several stages. Institutions first submit proposals to one of the state's seven regional planning councils, which review each application and make a recommendation to the New York State Hospital Review and Planning Council. The council, in turn, offers its recommendation to the Commissioner of Health, who has final authority to approve or disapprove the addition of new facilities and services in all cases except the establishment of new hospitals in the state. By the mid-1980s, New York had also developed "appropriateness review" standards for a wide range of clinical interventions and specialized services, including neonatal special care, acute-care beds, chronic dialysis, extracorporeal shockwave lithotripsy, hospital emergency departments, tuberculosis and AIDS beds, and cardiac surgery.

Even before the passage of Metcalf-McClosky, however, concerns over rising Blue Cross premiums prompted Governor Nelson Rockefeller to create a Committee on Hospital Costs to explore the rapid rise in hospital inflation in the early 1960s. The committee's report was released in 1965 and recommended that all state functions related to hospital regulation be consolidated within the Department of Health (DOH), which would be responsible for overseeing the activities of the state's hospital and nursing home industries (Somers 1969, 145–46). In addition to regulating hospital construction, the committee urged the DOH to establish a uniform reporting system for monitoring hospital costs, with detailed annual reports submitted to the DOH by each hospital. The report also proposed that "payments for hospital services by government agencies be at rates that are reasonably related to the costs of providing such services; [the previous year's] cost reports provide the basis for establishing reimbursement rates for the subsequent year" (Somers 1969, 167). By providing officials in the DOH with access to detailed cost and utilization information about institutional performance, the report laid the foundation for more extensive regulation of the hospital industry.

Additional pressure for state control of health care costs emerged after the passage of Medicare and Medicaid in 1965. Neither the legislature nor the governor fully appreciated the impact of Medicaid on New York's fiscal health. The enabling legislation that created New York's Medicaid program offered unusually generous eligibility standards: more than 45% of the state's population was eligible for benefits under the income limits approved by the legislature in 1966 (Stevens and Stevens 1973, 92). These terms approved by the legislature reflected the unique problem of providing care for the poor in New York City; the high cost of living in the city relative to rural and suburban communities elsewhere in the state necessitated a higher income threshold for city residents.

Governor Rockefeller's assumption that only a minority of eligible persons would sign up for Medicaid proved to be correct; by 1967 New York City began a door-to-door campaign to enroll welfare recipients and the "medically indigent" in the program (Stevens and Stevens 1974, 97). Costs soon exceeded even the most fiscally conservative estimates; actual program expenditures for FY1967 were 31% ($111 million) over budget. By 1968, New York faced a Medicaid-induced fiscal crisis as the state's share of program costs reached $426 million; amendments to the program signed into law by the Johnson administration in 1967 threatened to increase the state's contribution to both Aid to Families with Dependent Children (AFDC) and Medicaid by nearly $150 million. In the face of rampant inflation from both rising enrollments and provider charges, the legislature approved sweeping cuts in program eligibility—from $6,000 to $5,300 for a family of four. These changes were expected to save the state more than $300 million by sharply reducing the number of eligible beneficiaries (Stevens and

Stevens 1974, 163). Even with these alterations, however, New York's income eligibility criteria remained the most generous in the nation.

By the late 1960s, legislative concerns over rising Blue Cross premiums led to the passage of Chapter 957 in 1969, which mandated that Blue Cross pay providers on a prospective basis. Furthermore, since the act linked Blue Cross reimbursement rates to those of the state Medicaid program, more than half of hospital revenues were controlled by the DOH, which was empowered to use peer-group comparisons of institutional rates in order to encourage the "efficient" delivery of hospital services. The peer groups established by Chapter 957, however, effectively institutionalized existing differences in payment rates between "upstate" and "downstate" hospitals. These reforms, coupled with several "charge-control" bills passed during the state's fiscal crisis in the mid-1970s, established ceilings on reimbursable costs, limited allowable length of stay, and limited payment for outpatient services under Medicaid. These reforms, however, were largely incremental efforts to control the state's immediate fiscal problems.

More comprehensive efforts at reform would not come until 1978 when the legislature established the Council on Health Care Financing to plan for the introduction of an all-payer rate-setting system. The state's first all-payer system emerged out of discussions between the council and legislative leaders in 1982. The New York Prospective Hospital Reimbursement Methodology (NYPHRM), building on the system of charge controls for Blue Cross and Medicaid that had been in place since the early 1970s, paid hospitals on the basis of their costs per inpatient day.[2] Implementation of NYPHRM in the early 1980s severely restricted the financial autonomy of the state's acute-care hospitals by establishing fixed differentials among rates charged by third-party payers.[3] NYPHRM also placed a ceiling on the maximum amount hospitals could charge a patient, regardless of who was footing the bill, thereby limiting the opportunity for hospitals to recoup expenses disallowed by state regulators. While NYPHRM maintained the differential between Blue Cross and the charge payers established under the state's earlier rate-setting efforts, its magnitude was greatly reduced. The new pricing scheme was overtly designed to change the behavior of high-cost institutions by providing a strong fiscal incentive to provide care at a lower cost. In short, by the mid-1980s the incentives for health care providers in New York were determined by the state, not the market.

Although NYPHRM placed a number of restrictions on cost shifting, it also offered a carrot to the state's hospital industry with the addition of regional free care and bad debt pools funded by a surcharge on inpatient hospital rates.[4] Revenues from the surcharge were deposited into several regional pools which were allocated to hospitals according to their level of bad debt and charity care for the previous year. The creation of bad debt and free care pools was the state's first attempt to address the lingering concerns of hospitals about uncompensated care (e.g., services provided to indigent patients or services deemed uncollectible). While the Hill-Burton program required hospitals to furnish some free care in exchange for federal subsidies for hospital construction, hospitals had long argued that they should be reimbursed for the costs associated with providing such services.

NYPHRM remained in effect from 1983 to 1985, despite the passage of the federal government's new prospective-payment system (PPS) for Medicare in 1983. After the Medicare waiver expired on December 31, 1985, HCFA began paying hospitals in New York on the basis of diagnosis-related groups (DRGs) for all Medicare inpatient care. Before the waiver expired, however, the legislature enacted a new payment system (NYPHRM II) that continued the per diem reimbursement methodology for all payers except Medicare. NYPHRM II also created an assessment on hospital revenues to compensate for the federal government's reduced contributions to the regional free care and bad debt pools. The pools, however, were controlled by the Department of Health; funds were explicitly targeted to institutions treating a disproportionate share of the uninsured.

The hospital industry welcomed the end of the waiver because Medicare's PPS was considerably more generous in its reimbursements than NYPHRM's per diem methodology.[5] Office of Health Systems Management's (OHSM) Director of Hospital Reimbursement noted that the state "gave up the [HCFA] waiver because it was worth $400 million to the hospitals. I couldn't recommend to my principals that we not allow the hospitals a $400 million infusion of federal funds." In addition, the growing cost of physician malpractice insurance in the mid-1980s led the legislature to mandate that hospitals purchase malpractice coverage for their staff physicians. This requirement imposed a significant fiscal burden on many large teaching institutions with hundreds of physicians on staff.

NYPHRM II was conceived as a temporary solution to bridge the gap between the all-payer system, including Medicare, and the non-Medicare all-payer system. As such, it was an ad hoc creation which essentially carried forward the methodology introduced in 1983 with only minor modifications. After Medicare switched to a case-based payment system, however, state officials began actively investigating options for implementing a similar system in New York. Planning for a new case-based payment system began in 1986, nearly two years before the expiration of NYPHRM II. In 1988, the legislature embraced the recommendations of the Health Department and the Business

Council by establishing a case-based payment system (NYPHRM III) for all payers except Medicare.[6] Legislation to change the base year for NYPHRM III from 1981 to 1985 was vetoed by Governor Cuomo. As one senior official in the OHSM argued, the state opposed a change in the base year in 1988 because it wanted to "deal with the changes in the hospital payment system as targeted infusions into the base for a variety of public policy reasons."

Unlike Medicare's PPS, hospital reimbursement under NYPHRM III was based entirely on New York State hospital data trended forward from 1981. DRG-weights were also based on statewide rather than national experience, using data drawn from a sample of 90 hospitals for all non-Medicare patients. Hospital non-Medicare data were used to create a rate of payment, which was then adjusted by each third-party payer according to a pre-established set of rate differentials. NYPHRM III established a fixed differential between Blue Cross, Medicaid, and all other nongovernment payers.[7] The basic structure of the system remained unchanged after the legislature's renewal of the Empire State's case-based payment system in 1990 created NYPHRM IV. In particular, NYPHRM IV continued one of its predecessor's most controversial aspects in its use of group pricing to determine hospital reimbursement. Under NYPHRM III, hospitals were reimbursed partially on their own historical costs and partially on the average cost for a peer group of hospitals; the percentage of hospital revenues computed using the group average, or "pricing," component increased from 10% in 1988 to 55% in 1990. Despite the health department's urgings, the legislature balked at moving to a 100% group price, in which each hospital's reimbursement for a procedure would be based on the average price within its peer group. With no change in the base year planned, the case-based reimbursement system introduced in 1988 remained in place until December 1993, when the last iteration of the state's prospective-payment system was approved in the final days of the legislative session. Although the Department of Health developed a comprehensive proposal to create a single-payer financing system (dubbed "UNY*CARE") in the early 1990s, the effort failed to win enthusiastic support from either the governor's office or the legislature (Beauchamp 1993; Beauchamp and Rouse 1990).

NYPHRM IV expanded the use of pools to enable individuals to purchase care rather than subsidizing the provision of direct services by hospitals; after 1990, state subsidies for the Child Health Plus program were funded through the state's Bad Debt and Charity Care pools (Fraser 1995). NYPHRM IV also authorized the Department of Health to divert inpatient care funds to expand primary health services and required voluntary nonprofit hospitals to develop "community service plans" to address continuing problems of access to health care services.

As in previous iterations of the state's payment system, NYPHRM IV and its successor continued to emphasize targeted fiscal aid to distressed hospitals serving vulnerable populations through the use of regional pools. Both NYPHRM IV and NYPHRM V, however, were evolutionary refinements of the existing case-based payment methodology (Fraser 1995). Neither redefined the scope of state regulatory powers or challenged the basic premises of the state's approach to cost containment.

New York's rapidly rising expenditures on Medicaid in the early 1990s did not reflect a weakened commitment to cost containment but rather an opportunistic effort to exploit federal matching funds on the part of state officials. In recent years, many states have attempted to shift state-funded programs into Medicaid in order to qualify for federal matching funds (Coughlin et al. 1994). While New York began to move Medicaid beneficiaries into managed care after 1990 in an effort to control costs, the state also attempted to shift thousands of general assistance recipients funded exclusively by state and local governments into the federal SSI program in order to capture federal matching funds. In addition, the state shifted its bad debt and charity pools into Medicaid and imposed a provider tax on hospitals and nursing homes to increase Medicaid billings (Coughlin et al. 1994). Thus, while total Medicaid expenditures rose sharply from 1988 to 1992, transferring programs that had previously been 100% state funded into Medicaid or SSI enabled state officials to free up funds for other programs and/or expand services to program beneficiaries.

Over the past decade, New York has increasingly turned to managed care as a solution to controlling rising Medicaid costs. In 1982, HCFA approved the state's application for a Freedom of Choice demonstration waiver to implement a mandatory prepaid managed care program for all AFDC and general assistance ("Home Relief") beneficiaries in Monroe County. By 1986, more than 42,000 persons had been enrolled in the state's Medicaid Managed care waiver program. The state offered beneficiaries the opportunity to voluntarily enroll in prepaid health plans over the next decade. In 1991, the legislature mandated that all of the state's local social service departments develop a managed care program within five years, with the goal of enrolling more than 50% of the eligible popuation by 1996. By 1994, more than 26% of the state's 1.8 million Medicaid-eligibles were enrolled in prepaid health service plans or HMOs (New York State 1995). To date, however, final approval of the state's application for a Section 1115 demonstration waiver is still pending.

In 1995, the Pataki administration applied for a Section 1115 research and demonstration waiver to allow the state to mandate enrollment in managed care for 87% of the state's noninstitutionalized recipients. In its waiver application to HCFA, the state proposed to ensure that "each Medicaid recipient has a 'medical home' and a rational way to obtain health care services." In addition to mandating enrollment in managed care plans for eligible beneficiaries, New York's waiver application proposed to contract with "special needs plans" to provide fully capitated services to persons with HIV/AIDS, the mentally ill, and emotionally disturbed children.

After his election in November 1994, Governor George Pataki indicated that he would seek alternative options for controlling health care costs in New York State which relied on market incentives, not regulation. Since legislative authorization for NYPHRM V was scheduled to expire on June 30, 1996, the governor appointed an ad hoc task force chaired by Health Commissoner Barbara DeBuono to develop recommendations for reforming the state's health care financing system. The goals and operating assumptions of the new task force repudiated the regulatory approach to controlling health care costs, which had evolved over the previous decade. In their final report to the governor, members argued that their "principal mission is to shift the policy debate from discussions of mechanisms for hospital financing to approaches that promote a healthier New York" (New York Department of Health 1995b). To achieve this goal, the NYPHRM task force recommended that the state enact policies to "promote competition in the health care marketplace by increasing reliance on market incentives while reducing the role of regulation."

The task force endorsed moving from the current rate-setting system to one where providers would be free to negotiate their rates with all non-Medicare payers and Medicaid; the Department of Health, however, would be allowed to engage in selective contracting and negotiate Medicaid fee-for-service rates. The members of the task force justified their recommendations on the grounds that (1) negotiated rates would reduce excess capacity in the health care system by encouraging hospitals to "rightsize" their operations; (2) NYPHRM's fee-for-service method of reimbursement offered an incompatible set of incentives in a health care system with rising managed care penetration; and (3) since market forces were already "exerting economic pressure on the health care system," state regulation of hospital reimbursement was no longer necessary. The task force did, however, recognize the need for expanded subsidies for insurance coverage, the continuation of state funding for uncompensated care, and, in a signficant departure, also recommended that hospitals should negotiate financing for capital projects with third-party payers; under NYPHRM, capital projects were funded through surcharges on hospital inpatient and outpatient rates.

The deregulation plan passed by the Legislature in July 1996 (Chapter 639) closely followed the principles articulated in the ad hoc task force's final report. Although the Pataki administration and legislative leaders had reached a consensus that hospitals should be free to negotiate their own rates with third-party payers, funding for graduate medical education, uncompensated care, and capital financing remained in dispute throughout the 1996 legislative session (Dao 1996b). Under the compromise deregulation plan, state funding for graduate medical education fell from $1.9 billion in 1995 to $1.4 billion, financed by a surchage on health insurance policies, while a similar assessment on inpatient revenues provided $786 million for the state's Bad Debt and Charity Care pools (Dao 1996b). In addition, legislators remained committed to funding other "public goods" to increase access to health care; Chapter 639 continued the state's Child Health Plus insurance program to provide primary care and preventative services for low-income children and allocated more than $200 million per year for worker retraining, quality improvement, and the implementation of mandatory enrollment in Medicaid managed care plans.

The Success of Cost Containment in New York State

The fiscal condition of the state's hospitals, as measured by a variety of operating indicators, was among the weakest in the United States during the 1980s and 1990s (see Bentkover, Schroeder, and Lee 1985). New York and Alaska were the only two states that experienced negative operating margins for five consecutive years from 1988 to 1992 (Cleverly 1993, 21). In addition, New York's hospitals were considerably less liquid than their counterparts in other states; the median hospital in New York had only 11.07 days cash-on-hand in 1992, the lowest in the nation (Cleverly 1993, 67). In 1989, the average operating margin for hospitals in New York ranked forty-ninth in the nation, while the average total profit margin for the industry in the state came in fiftieth (Hospital Association of New York State 1990a). Furthermore, the state's stringent certificate-of-need review criteria in the 1970s and early 1980s left the Empire State with some of the nation's oldest health care facilities. The consequence of New York's restrictive system of regulatory controls has been a dramatic decline in the number of non-government hospitals (Thorpe 1989); more than ninety facilities closed their doors or were converted to others uses since the beginning of the state's fiscal crisis in 1975. As the number of acute-care facilities declined (from 329 in 1974 to 235 in 1992), the state's occupancy rate, already one of the nation's highest, increased from 83% to 87% over the same period.

The fiscal condition of the state's hospital industry is directly related to the restrictive planning and reimbursement practices introduced over the past three decades. As Mitchell (1988, 93) observes, New York's policies during the 1970s and 1980s reduced the growth of hospital spending more than any other state in the nation. By the end of the decade, the unmet need for hospital renovation and replacement exceeded two-thirds of the state's acute-care bed capacity (Mitchell 1988). The combined effect of rate-setting and certificate-of-need (CON) requirements over the past two decades has been a dramatic reduction in both the fiscal health and managerial autonomy of hospitals in New York State. After a string of operating losses in the 1980s and early 1990s, hospitals in New York reported modest profits in 1993 and 1994 (Bauder 1992; Denn 1994). Hospitals and the Department of Health, however, continue to spar over the appropriate methodology for assessing the industry's fiscal health; while state officials count charity and endowment income and revenue from real estate sales in their computations, hospitals focus on the operating surplus (or loss) from patient services (Bauder 1992). As a result, policymakers are routinely presented with conflicting reports of the industry's financial condition.

Both CON and rate-setting provided state officials with the means to restructure the delivery of health care services in New York. While the coordination of CON and rate-setting functions can be difficult due to differences in the goals and incentives of each (Kinney 1987), the centralization of regulatory authority within the Office of Health Systems Management ensured that both programs would reflect the state's interest in cost containment.

During the early 1980s, the Department of Health imposed a moratorium on the construction of new hospital beds, based upon econometric studies from the Division of Health Facility Planning that projected a surplus of more than 18,000 acute-care beds by 1990. While many hospitals closed their doors during the late 1980s, the state was still projecting a surplus of beds by 1989. By the end of the decade, however, the deteriorating condition of aging hospital physical plants led to a more accommodative stance toward construction and renovation proposals by the State Hospital Review and Planning Council. By the early 1990s, New York City was experiencing a hospital construction boom, as several institutions received approval to replace aging physical plants or upgrade facilities. After more than a decade in which new hospital construction was strongly discouraged, one regional hospital association president argued that "what we're seeing now is replacement and renovation that had been held up for a number of years. This is basically catch up" (quoted in Dunlap 1993). The disposition of CON applications by the State Hospital Review and Planning Council supports this view: the denial rate for CON proposals fell considerably from the mid-1980s to the early 1990s (see Tables 3.1 and 3.2).

Despite its stringent review thresholds and the imposition of a moratorium on the construction of new acute-care beds, hospitals had discovered several loopholes in the statutory framework of the CON

TABLE 3.1 Disposition of CON Applications: Acute-Care Facilities*

Year	Approved (%)	Denied (%)	N
1985	43 (100)	0 (0)	43
1986	36 (80)	9 (20)	45
1987	87 (100)	0 (0)	87
1988	111 (85)	19 (15)	130
1989	70 (89)	9 (11)	79
1990	54 (93)	4 (7)	58
1991	64 (99)	1 (1)	65
1992	75 (100)	0 (0)	75
1993	72 (94)	5 (6)	77
Total:	612 (93)	47 (7)	659

Source: *CON Annual Reports,* 1982–93, New York Department of Health, Division of Health Facility Planning. Data computed from material in Table II, "Analysis of applications recommended for approval/disapproval by the state council by type of proposal."

*Includes all proposals for major modernization projects, the addition of acute-care hospital beds, nonmedical equipment, minor renovations, and minor service changes.

process in New York by the mid-1970s. Since physicians and other noninstitutional health care providers were not subject to CON review for the first two decades of the program's operation, some institutions circumvented restrictions on the acquisition of new technology by encouraging staff radiologists to purchase and operate CT scanners in adjacent buildings (Roos 1987, 511–12). Other strategies included acquiring equipment in a piecemeal fashion to keep the price of components below the review threshold, cooperative ventures with physicians who owned the equipment and leased it back to the hospital, and the use of corporate subsidiaries to apply for CON approval. In stark contrast to legal challenges against the state's reimbursement system, hospitals in New York have successfully appealed unfavorable CON rulings to the courts (Roos 1987).

The Department of Health has actively promoted the conversion of acute-care hospital beds to meet growing demand for specialized services over the past decade (e.g., AIDS, tuberculosis, traumatic brain injury), but the CON process in New York appears less effective in controlling the diffusion of new technologies than in constricting the

TABLE 3.2   Disposition of CON Applications: Medical Equipment

Year	Approved (%)	Denied (%)	N
1985	40 (100)	0 (0)	40
1986	32 (89)	4 (11)	36
1987	27 (100)	0 (0)	27
1988	64 (85)	11 (15)	75
1989	24 (92)	2 (8)	24
1990	11 (85)	2 (15)	13
1991	25 (96)	1 (4)	26
1992	24 (100)	0 (0)	24
1993	18 (100)	0 (0)	18
Total:	265 (93)	20 (7)	285

Source: *CON Annual Reports*, 1985–93, New York Department of Health, Division of Health Facility Planning. Data computed from material in Table II, "Analysis of applications recommended for approval/disapproval by the state council by type of proposal."

bed supply. In part, this is a function of the program's statutory design, for the Empire State's low review threshold "spawns efforts on the part of health care facilities and physicians to circumvent the literal requirements" (Roos 1987, 518–19). By the early 1990s, the effects of the state's moratorium on renovation and new construction during the previous decade were evident, as New York hospitals operated some of the oldest physical plants in the nation. The demonstrated need for the replacement or renovation of several major teaching hospitals fueled a statewide construction boom as the state Hospital Review and Planning Council approved more than $6 billion in construction in New York City alone over a three-year period (Dunlap 1993).

THE NATURE OF THE DECISION-MAKING PROCESS IN NEW YORK STATE

The relationship between the state and societal interests moved through several distinct phases over the past three decades. In each phase, however, state officials set the terms of the regulatory policy agenda and when needed enlisted the support of business groups or third-party payers to further the state's interest in cost containment. While New York's persistent fiscal crises have provided the motive for state intervention, the institutional capacity of the state's policy-making institutions has strengthened the ability of public officials to overcome intense opposition from health care providers. Health care policy-making in New York over the past two decades has been defined by a "strong state" (Krasner 1978), pursuing policies which are inimical to powerful societal actors. In particular, the implementation of restrictive reimbursement policies in New York were designed to control costs, minimize cost shifting, and subsidize the provision of care to the indigent and "high-risk" populations. Although each of these goals drew the ire of health care providers and third-party payers, the legitimacy of state authority to regulate the health care industry has withstood frequent legal challenges in state and federal courts.

Imposed regulatory regimes are characterized by a high degree of cohesion among key policymakers. The central role of cost containment as a goal for state health policy has been accepted by state officials, third-party payers, and business groups. Although health care providers—and hospitals in particular—have contested public officials' definitions of both the means and ends of state cost-containment policies, price regulation, utilization controls, and health planning have enjoyed bipartisan support since the 1960s. The policy image (Baumgartner and Jones 1991) of health care costs as a threat to the state's fiscal stability and economic competitiveness has defined the context of health care policy-making in New York since the late 1950s.

The precise definition of the problem, however, has changed over time. In the 1950s and 1960s, the "cost crisis" was defined by concerns about the rising cost of health insurance premiums. By the late 1960s, however, Medicaid had emerged as the principal object of cost-control concerns as rising expenditures on health care for the poor left legislators in a politically untenable position; in the face of soaring program costs, lawmakers could either raise taxes, cut eligibility, or restrict payments to providers. By the mid-1980s, however, health care cost containment was also viewed as an economic development tool, for the high cost of doing business in the state had resulted in a mass exodus of firms into Connecticut and New Jersey.

The political viability of extensive regulation of the hospital industry in New York State is linked to the state's commitment to expansive social programs. In 1993, New York's Medicaid program accounted for 16% of total program expenditures nationwide (Denn 1995). In general, New York has exhibited a "bipartisan commitment to high government expenditures, high taxes, and state-mandated public service programs" in recent decades (Liebschutz and Lurie (1987, 169). By all accounts, New York has a liberal political culture that crosses party lines, a characteristic evident in both survey-based and policy-based measures (Erikson, Wright, and McIver 1985). Measures of state-policy liberalism place New York as the most liberal state in the nation (Holbrook-Provow and Poe 1987, 406). The expanded role for the public sector is particularly clear in state rankings of per capita expenditures and revenues relative to other states. New York's per capita spending on elementary and secondary education, welfare, health and hospitals, and the overall level of state general expenditures were among the highest in the nation during the 1980s and 1990s (Colby and White 1989, 236). In this context, extensive regulation of health care providers in New York served an instrumental purpose, for price controls enabled the state to provide expanded services without experiencing chronic deficits.

Most reforms prior to the late 1970s were designed to bring the Empire State's Medicaid budget under control. Following the creation of the state's Medicaid program in 1966, rampant cost inflation provided the rationale for the state's first rate-setting efforts in 1969 and legitimated subsequent expansions of rate review to all payers in the 1970s and 1980s. The passage of Chapter 76 in 1976, however, underscored the state's compelling interest in cost control. The legislature authorized the Commissioner of Health to promulgate "necessary rules and regulations," set payment rates, and control inpatient hospital utilization and length of stay. Legislators also froze Medicaid payments at FY1975 levels through March 1977 and empowered the Commissioner to "suspend, limit, or revoke a general hospital operating certificate, after taking into consideration the total number of beds necessary to meet the public need."

Both the restrictions on hospital reimbursment and the extraordinary expansion of the Department of Health's control over the internal management and operations of private hospitals were a direct response to the state's fiscal crisis. Indeed, with the passage of Chapter 76, legislators noted that "state and local governments are facing fiscal crises of staggering proportions and cannot continue to support the scope and level of assistance, care, and services, the cost of which has sharply escalated in recent years." Spurred on by fiscal crisis, the state legislature granted the Department of Health broad regulatory powers to control health care costs. As one regional hospital association president argued, "The state's philosophy is to maintain control over its programs so that it can handle its budgetary problems." In retrospect, the Omnibus Budget Reconciliation Act in 1981 "buttressed the activist interventionist traditions of New York State government. . . . Reductions in federal funding under Reagan . . . resulted in greater state centralization in the Empire State" (Liebschutz and Lurie 1987, 170).

The state's rule-making authority sparked heated debate over the fairness of the system and repeated charges of "micromanagement" by hospital industry representatives during the 1980s. From the industry's perspective, the Department of Health's rule-making powers had become so extensive that the department was no longer accountable for its actions. According to Dan Sisto, the president of the Hospital Association of New York State, the state's regulatory system "needs to differentiate the payers from the regulators. I have no objection to state government performing those functions, but I think some separation of those powers might be necessary because what is emerging is a hospital system whose financing is dependent on the state budget, but whose performance expectations are cast at levels unobtainable because of that budget" (quoted in Gustis 1989, E5). State officials challenged this view, arguing that "what we have in New York is a system where the primary concern is not the patient. We have an entitlement program for providers" (quoted in Denn 1995).

In the early years of state regulation, 1960–68, Fox (1991, 734) argues that Blue Cross "enlisted New York State as its ally in controlling the growth of capital expenditures." State officials, however, were the driving force behind the creation of New York's health planning initiatives in the mid-1960s, for where state and societal preferences are nondivergent, public officials may implement their own preferences as policy (Nordlinger 1981). The state's foray into health planning was supported by both hospitals and Blue Cross, but each had very different reasons for endorsing certificate-of-need and regional planning. Blue Cross favored facilities regulation in the belief that controlling the construction of new facilities and the introduction of new technologies would help to control spiraling premium growth; hospitals, for their part, viewed the proposed planning statute as a less intrusive alternative to rate regulation.

At the time, state officials were principally interested in preserving the affordability of Blue Cross coverage, for the Kerr-Mills program was not a significant drain on the state budget. Furthermore, while Blue Cross officials embraced the notion of planning and capital expenditure review, they were reluctant to challenge the prerogatives of health care providers directly by negotiating more advantageous terms of reimbursement. While some critics (Law 1976) have argued that the development of New York's certificate-of-need and health planning programs reflects the ability of Blue Cross to persuade the state to control its costs through the use of public authority, such an interpretation neglects the role of state officials in expanding the state's regulatory powers (Marmor 1991, 778–79).

State autonomy expanded considerably in the years following the passage of Medicaid. Beginning in 1969, legislators and the governor turned to rate setting as the principal lever to bring Medicaid costs under control. The Blues also supported state regulation, but the company role after 1969 changed from a coequal partner with the state to a supportive constituent group, for Medicaid costs were the principal impetus behind changes in the health care financing system during the 1970s and 1980s. Hospitals did not seriously challenge the introduction of rate-setting in New York, despite considerable reservations about ceding authority over health care financing to the state. In the face of a Medicaid-induced fiscal crisis, the legislature proposed a freeze on Medicaid reimbursement rates (Stevens and Stevens 1974). Although this action was later held to be unconstitutional, hospitals viewed rate-setting as the lesser of two evils in 1969 and acquiesced to the state's expanded regulatory authority.

On many occasions, however, the policy preferences of public officials diverge sharply from those of the hospital industry and, in several cases, of commercial insurers and HMOs. The controversy over new hospital operating standards, in particular, provides a clear example of what Nordlinger (1981) defines as "type I state autonomy," where the decisions of state officials are "contrary to the demands of any private actors, including the best endowed actors who predominate consistently within civil society, and [they] do so with some frequency" (Nordlinger 1981, 118). The pricing policies of the Department of Health during the 1980s provide numerous examples of such actions. Department officials emphasized that the flow of funds to the hospital industry remained a public policy question that must be decided by the state, rather than by private markets. As Health Commissioner Axelrod noted in 1989, "There will be new money [for the hospitals]; there has to be. We are dealing with an increasingly vulnerable population. But the way in which we spend it will be much more carefully scrutinized. There will be continuing concern about the equity in the allocation of resources" (quoted in Gustis 1989, E5).

Few opportunities exist for close collaboration between the hospital industry and the state on pricing issues in the Empire State. Indeed, hospital industry officials contend that the DOH is not interested in working together at all. As one HANYS official recounted in 1990,

> There's no state health policy in this state. If you interviewed the top brightest people in this state, the only thing that would emerge would be "let's screw down the hospitals." There's no collaboration. [Commissioner Axelrod] becomes sort of a lightning rod for this. I said to him once, "let's get beyond these troubled waters and look at things five or ten years out." His response was "I'm very fond of you personally, but I don't have any interest in collaborating with the hospital industry in this state." After about an hour and a half of that, I walked away and said to myself that there are not too many places where the level of adversarialism has gotten to the point where there's only one way of looking at the truth.

Nor was Axelrod's rhetoric designed to mollify industry critics; in speeches to the business community, he referred to the hospitals as "seventeenth-century Germanic guilds." Under these circumstances, as one HANYS executive quipped, "it's tough to get people to be statesmanlike."

The relative isolation of hospitals in the policy process is clear in the development of new policy initiatives within the Department of Health. As one OHSM staffer observed in 1990, ideas for new programs "come in from the legislature, the Commissioner, [and] from our own initiatives." Notably absent from this list are representatives from the hospital industry and third-party payers. Indeed, HANYS' officials contend that most decisions are arrived at without consulting those groups which are most affected until the formal hearings mandated under the rule-making process.

The desire of state officials to exercise control over the allocation of resources in the hospital industry is illustrated by two of the more controversial issues between the department and health care providers in the 1980s and early 1990s: moving the base year for the payment system and the selective infusion of additional funds to the industry. Hospital reimbursement rates were updated annually by a calculated trend factor designed to account for changes in input prices over the past fiscal year. The hospital industry, however, contended that the computation of the trend factor was inherently unfair since the base year for all computations remained unchanged after New York moved to its all-payer system in 1981. Officials in the Department of Health took a very different position on the matter. For the department, changing the base year involved more than merely readjusting the basis of comparisons from 1981 to a more recent year. Since the financial positions, case mixes, and payer mixes of institutions seldom remain the same over time, new peer groups must also be devised to reflect these changes. In a worst-case scenario, an institution could find itself moved from a peer group where its costs were average or below average to one where its cost per case exceeded the group average. This is not an improbable scenario, particularly for hospitals with large AIDS caseloads. Since hospitals were paid a flat rate per case under the DRG system, an institution's financial position in these circumstances could change from profitability to an operating deficit virtually overnight. As one senior official in OHSM pointed out,

> One of the reasons we have not moved the base year is that we have tried to deal with changes in the hospital reimbursement system as targeted infusions into the base for a variety of public policy reasons. . . . Hospitals have a very pluralistic revenue stream, and that revenue stream will drive

them to do very different things beyond what we would put in as a reasonable trend factor. . . . Certain institutions don't have these pluralistic revenue streams so you've got have and have-not issues [and] . . . our position has been that infusions into the system should be targeted to produce a more level playing field. . . . As you get farther away from it [the 1981 base], it becomes less and less of an issue because you're really on a revenue stream as opposed to a cost stream.[8]

Differences over the base year and hospital dissatisfaction with the department's policy of selectively targeting additional funds into the reimbursement system reflect the activist philosophy internalized by state officials within the DOH. Despite the persistence of fundamental tensions between the department and the hospital industry, policymakers within OHSM have not wavered from their aggressive pursuit of cost control over the past two decades. The department's approach to cost containment reflects an emphasis on directing the behavior of nonprofit organizations to achieve public purposes. As the OHSM's director of hospital reimbursement observed in 1990, New York's regulatory policies reflected the ideas of Robert Anthony and Regina Herzlinger, who argued that

Prices should be equal to full costs. . . . The rationale for full cost pricing is as follows: A nonprofit organization often has a monopoly position. It should not set prices that exceed its cost, for to do so would take advantage of its monopoly status. Furthermore, the organization does not need to price above cost. If it does so, it generates a profit, and by definition no person can benefit from such a profit (Anthony and Herzlinger 1980, 387).

The institutional capacities of state government in New York have few rivals. Albany became a hub of activity as both the size of state government and the scope of state regulatory powers expanded steadily after the 1950s. In particular, each of the principal public players in health care financing—the legislature, the governor, and the Department of Health—developed expansive formal powers and administrative expertise in health care policy-making. Policymakers' efforts to fashion solutions to New York's pressing fiscal problems in the 1970s and 1980s were bolstered by the growing administrative capacity and policy-making coherence of state political institutions. Controlling Medicaid costs through regulation enjoyed strong bipartisan support from legislators, the governor's office, and local governments in New York, for Medicaid had contributed to a fiscal crisis for both the state and for local governments, which contributed between 10 and 25% of the program's operating budget.

Over the past three decades, the staggering cost of Medicaid in New York has provided the rationale for the development of a comprehensive set of regulatory controls over the hospital industry. The state's Medicaid program is unmatched in size and cost: New York spends more on Medicaid than any other state in the nation, nearly double the national average per capita (Denn 1995). Furthermore, growth in program costs averaged nearly 11% a year over the past decade (New York State 1995). In short, the Medicaid program in New York has created a state of perpetual fiscal crisis in Albany.

The Legislature

In New York, as elsewhere, the attractiveness of legislative service has increased steadily over the years, and concurrently, the power and influence of the legislature relative to other branches of government have increased as well. As Fowler and McClure's (1989, 76) discussion of legislative recruitment illustrates, "Over the past two decades, New York's state legislature has become a career-oriented institution that offered its senior members high salaries and enough electoral security, staff, and personal influence to make service in Albany increasingly competitive with service in Washington." These changes are reflected in declining rates of turnover and retirement in both the Senate and Assembly. Annual retirement from both houses fell from more than 15% in 1964 to roughly 6% in 1984, while legislative salaries rose more than 250% over the same period (Fowler and McClure 1989). With a base salary of $57,500 for members of both chambers in 1994, New York legislators were the most highly paid state lawmakers in the nation (Council of State Governments 1994).[9]

The growing institutionalization of the state legislature in New York was evident in the aftermath of the 1994 elections, as turnover in both the Senate (3.3%) and the Assembly (9.3%) was among the lowest in the U.S. During the early 1970s, the staff assigned to the state legislature—and to legislative leaders in particular—became increasingly professionalized in both houses. Individual members enjoy the services of year-round staff in Albany and in their home districts. Key leaders in the Assembly and the Senate supported the move in recognition of a growing need for reliable information to address the increasing complexity of policy issues (Hevesi 1975, 58–59). In addition, legislative leaders also significantly increased the number of analysts and policy specialists assigned to key committees such as the Assembly Ways and Means Committee and the Senate Finance Committee; by 1980, each committee had a full-time staff of more than forty budget analysts and economists (Zimmerman 1981). The problem-solving capacities of legislators were also bolstered by the creation of a Central Staff Office for Assembly committees in 1970, which assigned teams of researchers to each committee chair as a supplement to his or her own staff (Hevesi 1975, 59). In 1980, the combined employment of the Assembly and Senate exceeded 3,000 professional staff, lawyers, and policy analysts (Zimmerman 1981). As in Washington (Arnold 1990), the members elected to the New York legislature during the 1970s and 1980s were "younger, more aggressive, better educated, more highly motivated, and definitely more productive and serious than their predecessors" (Hevesi 1989, 167).

By the mid-1970s, divided government had replaced the former pattern of Republican dominance in New York; the 1982 redistricting solidified Democratic control over the Assembly. Republicans, however, have controlled the Senate since 1965. Party competition and party voting are also high in both chambers. While the Democratic margin in the Assembly increased from 92–56 in 1986 to 96–52 in 1996, Republicans maintained solid control over the Senate in both 1986 (36–25) and 1996 (35–26). As Ciangrelli (1993, 256–57) noted,

> During the legislative process, Democrats almost automatically oppose Republican initiatives, and Republicans vote against Democratic proposals, unless there is some really good reason to do otherwise. . . . Partisanship is maintained by regular meetings of the four party caucuses, where vote tallies that for all practical purposes bind members on floor votes are taken. When party leaders go to the floor on issues, the outcome is almost always certain.

Coalition-building in the legislature is difficult due to intense conflicts between the interests of rural communities and smaller cities "upstate" versus "downstate" representatives from the New York City metropolitan area. The upstate/downstate cleavage, however, complements the legislature's existing party alignments, for over the past three decades New York City and the state's other major urban areas have been traditional Democratic bastions, while suburban and rural communities remained Republican strongholds (Ciangrelli 1993, 255–56). As a result, "For years, the dominant coalition in New York state politics has been between the governor and the Speaker of the Assembly against the majority leader of the Republican-controlled Senate" (Ciangrelli 1993, 257).

Power is highly centralized in both chambers of the New York State legislature. The Assembly Speaker controls appointments to standing committees, refers bills to committee, and serves as the chair of the Rules Committee. In addition, the Speaker assigns all personal staff to members and can delay action on bills until late in the legislative session, effectively ending their chance of passage (Zimmerman 1981, 129–30). The power of the leadership was particularly evident during the debate over the FY1997 budget and the Pataki administration's proposed hospital deregulation plan. As the July 4th holiday recess approached, Assembly Speaker Sheldon Silver and Senate Majority Leader Joseph L. Bruno informed legislators that a budget deal was imminent, but rank-and-file members had little idea of what was contained in the final accord (Hernandez 1996). One Assembly member described decision-making in the legislature as a "totally dysfunctional process. We're probably closer to the 1957 Bulgarian parliament than we are to a modern state legislature. We're stuck with Soviet-style politics in this place" (quoted in Hernandez 1996). Others legislators adopted a more moderate view of the process; one acknowledged that "the disadvantage of a strong legislative leadership is that the rank-and-file members don't play as big a role in the process" (quoted in Hernandez 1996). Legislative leaders exercised nearly complete control over the policy agenda in both chambers; in the closing hours of the 1996 legislative session, "newly printed bills were rushed to the floors of the Senate and Assembly so quickly that lobbyists and even some lawmakers had trouble getting copies before voting began" (Dao 1996c).

The Governor

Chief executives in New York State have historically dominated the legislative process, for the formal powers of the governor's office are considerable. Governors may call the legislature into special sessions whose agenda is limited to the issues defined by the executive branch. Recent occupants of the governor's office have shown an unusual fondness for their veto powers; from 1959 to 1974, Governor Nelson Rockefeller routinely vetoed more than 20% of the bills submitted to him by the legislature. In addition, the legislature has found it exceedingly difficult to override gubernatorial vetoes, most of which occur in a thirty-day postadjournment period following the end of the legislative session (Zimmerman 1981). Divided party control over the legislature also strengthens the governor's hand in policy-making, as few override attempts can gather sufficient support in both chambers.

Like his predecessors, Governor Cuomo was a leader in articulating New York's health policy agenda. In the words of one senior health department official, "He's been very active [on health policy issues]. . . . In the past year he held forums with hospital personnel in his office about hospital claims about not getting enough money [from the reimbursement system]." Cuomo's 1990 veto of the renewal of the state's case-based hospital payment system, which he viewed as inflationary, also illustrated his commitment to cost control. The payment bill was subsequently renegotiated with his personal involvement.

The administration of Governor George Pataki has also been actively involved in health care policy-making, albeit with a very different policy agenda than its precedessor. After defeating Cuomo's bid for re-election in 1994, Pataki set about selling his vision of a leaner and more entrepreneurial government for New York. "Whether it's welfare, Medicaid, or public housing, the whole idea should be not 'We're the government, we'll take care of you.' The idea should be 'You are a citizen in our society, and we want you to succeed'" (quoted in Traub 1996). Although he had inherited a $4.7 billion deficit from his predecessor, Pataki proposed sweeping program cuts as well as tax reductions as means to improve the state's economic competitiveness.

Legislators soon discovered that the new governor was willing to play hardball in order to achieve his objectives; during his first year in office, Pataki withheld the paychecks of legislators and their staff members in an effort to resolve an impasse over the state budget (Traub 1996). During the contentious negotiations over the state budget in 1996, Pataki threatened to allow the authorization for the state's hospital payment system to expire. Without an extension, hospitals faced a 12% cut in Medicaid payments, which industry groups described as "a tiger on the loose in the hospital community" that could "wreak enormous devastation" (Dao 1996a). To complicate matters further, negotiations over the deregulation of the hospital industry were linked by Governor Pataki to an ongoing dispute over rent controls in New York City; the Pataki administration sought concessions from "downstate" legislators as a price for supporting changes in the health care financing bill that would bolster the fiscal health of the city's teaching hospitals. In response to the governor's tactics, an unlikely coalition of downstate legislators, hospital industry lobbyists, and Republican lawmakers pressed the leadership to negotiate a deal with the administration. Once legislative protections for loft residents were resolved, a final bill to deregulate the state's hospital payment system passed in the waning hours of the 1996 legislative session.

The Bureaucracy

While decision-making responsibility for hospital reimbursement issues has shifted to the legislature over the past two decades, the implementation and administration of the state's rate-setting system still rests with the state Department of Health (DOH), and its efforts to control health care costs have enjoyed strong support from the governor's office in New York for more than three decades. The DOH was one of the first state agencies to employ a lobbyist to advance its agenda with key legislators in the 1960s and to work as a "departmental ambassador within the executive branch" (Hevesi 1975, 191). During the tenure of Dr. Andrew Fleck, the DOH's first intra-governmental lobbyist, the department began to develop its own legislative agenda, set priorities, lobby for bills, and enlist the support of external actors to advance its goals (Hevesi 1975, 191–92).

Within the DOH, rate-setting activities are concentrated in the Office of Health Systems Management (OHSM), created in 1977 as part of an administrative reorganization to centralize the Department's regulatory activities. At first glance, the most striking characteristic of OHSM's regulatory structure during the early 1990s was not its considerable size, but rather the experience of its senior management team. In 1990, all of the deputy directors, and most of the assistant directors in each OHSM division, had at least five years of policy-making experience with the department on health care financing issues. In several cases, key personnel had ten or more years of experience with the department (Hackey 1993a). Top policymakers within the DOH exhibited strong careerist sentiments over the past two decades. As one senior official at OHSM observed, working for the DOH "isn't a revolving door at all, and I think the reason for that is that the state has very competitive salaries; you make more dough here and the benefits are better."

The "revolving door" that often characterizes the staffing of regulatory agencies (Wilson 1980) was noticeably absent in the regulation of health care costs in New York during the 1980s and 1990s. For the state, the professionalization of expertise within the DOH and the legislature provided the foundation for the successful development and implementation of an increasingly complex system of regulatory controls. Since the department tends to promote from within, the actual number of senior officials leaving the department is quite low. In the opinion of the hospital industry, this is a major stumbling block. In the words of the president of one regional hospital association, the "senior people in DOH have been there for much too long. There's very little turnover there . . . they are the system." While stability is a drawback from the perspective of hospitals, it is a tremendous asset to the capacity of DOH to manage an exceptionally complex reimbursement system.

The prominence of the Department of Health in health care policy-making in New York was solidified during David Axelrod's twelve-year tenure as Commissioner of Health. At the time of his untimely departure from the department in 1991, Axelrod had served in his post longer than almost any agency head in state government (Sack 1991). While Axelrod's acerbic relationship with the state's hospital industry was legendary, his most enduring legacy continues to be the remarkable scope of regulatory powers he carved out for the department. His personal style (or lack thereof) "alienated virtually every constituency" (Vibbert 1991) in the state's health care policy-issue network at one point or another, and yet under his leadership the department established the most stringent hospital operating requirements in the nation, reformed medical education, fought vigorously to preserve the state's regional health planning agencies, and oversaw the development of the nation's most heavily regulated health care financing system. "Axelrod was widely believed to be the most powerful agency head in the Cuomo administration, personally close to the governor, and one of the few commissioners who saw Cuomo on a regular basis and talked with him frequently on the phone" (Beauchamp 1991, 204). His leadership and the strong support he enjoyed from the governor's office under both Hugh Carey and Mario Cuomo propelled the Department of Health to the forefront of health policy-making in New York. Indeed, as one state official recalled, "Cuomo's health policy has always been Axelrod's policy" (quoted in Sack 1991, B7).

In the late 1980s, the department's relationship with hospitals deteriorated further as Commissioner Axelrod pushed reforms in hospital operating standards to improve supervision of residents and interns in the state's teaching hospitals, limited the number of hours attending physicians and residents could work, and began a systematic study of the appropriateness of cardiac surgery. As the number of prepaid health plans operating in the state increased steadily during the 1980s, the commissioner warned providers that "we are going to make certain that those individuals who are enrolled in HMOs from different socioeconomc classes get the same care as anyone else" (quoted in Dana 1986). Under his leadership, New York also became the first state in the nation to implement a regional case-payment system which linked institutional reimbursement rates to patient outcome measures (New York State Department of Health 1990). Each of these actions either imposed significant costs upon the hospital industry, reduced the autonomy of administrators, or threatened to restrict the utilization of profitable services. All were consistent, however, with the department's efforts to redefine the organization and delivery of health care services in New York State.

The loss of David Axelrod to a debilitating stroke in 1991 removed the Department of Health's most forceful and effective advocate from state government. The search for a replacement left the department rudderless, as two budget cycles passed before the appointment of a new commissioner. After a lengthy confirmation process, Dr. Marc Chassin succeeded Axelrod as Commissioner of Health in 1992. Prior to joining the department, Chassin had established a national reputation as a pioneer in research on patient outcomes and the appropriate use of high technology services. Under his leadership, the department remained committed to cost containment but displayed a heightened interest in improving the quality and cost effectiveness of health care services. The new commissioner's technocratic leadership style, however, was a marked departure from that of his predecessor. Unlike Axelrod, Chassin pursued collaboration, not confrontation, with the hospital industry (Precious 1992). Patient advocacy groups noted that the new commissioner was "more of a team player" who was "not out there sparring all the time with hospitals, physicians, and the establishment" (quoted in Karlin 1993). Others offered less generous assessments of the commissioner's performance; in the eyes of the New York Public Interest Research Group, Chassin did "not seem to have the will to stand up to the medical establishment when they are wrong." Doctors, for their part, praised the new administration for "extend[ing] an olive branch" to providers (quoted in Karlin 1993).

Soon after the election of George Pataki in 1994, Chassin tendered his resignation. Barbara DeBuono, the former Director of Health in Rhode Island, was selected to replace Chassin in February 1995. During DeBuono's tenure, the emphasis of the state's cost-containment strategy soon shifted from regulation to promoting competition in the health care system. The new commissioner's health care reform task force forged a consensus on a plan to replace NYPHRM with a system of negotiated hospital rates while preserving state funding for uncompensated care and graduate medical education.

From top to bottom, the behavior of public officials in New York's Office of Health Systems Management over the past two decades was guided by a coherent and powerful set of role orientations and ideological beliefs. Top policymakers in the Office of Health Systems Management adopted and internalized a set of strong principles that guided their behavior in hospital financing matters. Many senior officials in OHSM had professional training as health economists and espoused a firm commitment to the desirability of cost-based pricing as the best means to achieve efficiency in the delivery of hospital services.[10] OHSM's Director of Hospital Reimbursement noted that "our focus in our [econometric] models is trying to move to patient-oriented systems, which basically means defining the physician-patient encounter and pricing it."

The OHSM has exhibited an unwavering commitment to controlling the cost of health care, particularly inpatient hospital care, since its creation in 1977. One senior OHSM manager contended that

Cost control is an integral part [of our mission] and has such a fiscal impact on the state's budget. It's been that way since 1968 and was really exacerbated by the fiscal crisis of 1976 and it continues to be a priority. . . . All non-Medicare payers are coupled because we're trying to keep the highest degree of leverage on this pluralistic system.

The department's agenda reflects an intense commitment to promoting the "efficient delivery of services" in the health sector. During the 1980s and early 1990s, OHSM officials expressed doubt that, left to their own devices, most hospitals would price their services on a competitive basis or provide adequate care to financially unattractive patients. The Department's Director of Hospital Reimbursement argued in 1990 that "Pricing for us is a measure of efficiency and it's a standard. Philosophically, why shouldn't a patient be paying the same for a coronary bypass in Albany as you would in New York City if we adjust appropriately for labor cost differentials?"

The Health Department opposed untargeted infusions of new funds into the payment system in the 1980s and 1990s on the grounds that resources should be targeted to areas of greatest need rather than being widely distributed among all acute-care hospitals. Furthermore, senior OHSM officials argued that upon close examination, the fiscal plight of many hospitals in New York could be traced to differences in managerial effectiveness, not excessive regulation. As one bureau director noted,

You've got hospitals on Long Island making $6 million and hospitals in New York City making money right down the road from hospitals that lose money. They can be 30 blocks apart, so you have to ask yourself the question: "Is it the payment system's fault?" I'm convinced that it's not the payment system itself. My objective is to try to not pay for hospitals but to pay for the services that it costs to treat patients. That's my goal. Are we fairly paying for the cost of patient care? That's my issue. Hospitals always worry about facility attributes, [but] the system is a cost-based system, so if you're breaking even, you're doing fairly well as a voluntary hospital . . . and if you're making money, I scratch my head and wonder on whose back you're making it.

TENSIONS WITHIN NEW YORK STATE'S HEALTH POLICY REGIME

A combination of internal contradictions, legal challenges, and shifting ideological tides contributed to the erosion of New York's State's imposed health policy regime during the 1990s. The passage of Chapter 639 of the New York Public Laws of 1996 marked the end of an era in state policy-making, for both the legislature and the governor effectively repudiated regulatory controls as a means of controlling health care costs. After twenty-five years of rate-setting, New York's health care system embraced deregulation, demonstrating that even highly institutionalized regulatory systems remain vulnerable to shifting economic and political winds. As with previous state efforts to control health care costs, however, deregulation won bipartisan support. The end of regulatory controls cannot be explained simply in terms of the triumph of conservatism, for after the Democratic leadership in the Assembly endorsed the broad outlines of the administration's reform plan in 1996, the final outcome was no longer in doubt. Instead, debate in the legislature focused on the technical details of implementation, particularly regarding funding for graduate medical education and other "public goods."

The demise of rate-setting in New York was the result of several underlying factors, each of which undermined the legitimacy of the existing regime. New York offers an example of regime change, for the underlying assumptions and goals of public policy shifted dramatically from 1990 to 1996. The extent of the transformation is striking. At the beginning of the decade, the policy-making climate in New York continued to support the expansion of state regulatory powers; the Department of Health's UNY*Care plan rested upon a strategy of "interposing a single payer between third-party payers and providers. UNY*Care will set rates for all providers and act as the single payer for all hospitals, physicians, clinics, and nursing homes" (New York State Department of Health 1990a, 6). Although never implemented, the Department's proposal won the endorsement of Governor Cuomo; a regional version of the model "electronic claims clearinghouse" was approved as a demonstration project by the Robert Wood Johnson Foundation. In short, all factors appeared to point to a growing state role in health care financing (Beauchamp 1993). Beneath the surface of the state's policy debates, however, underlying structural changes were weakening the effectiveness of NYPHRM's existing regulatory controls.

Changes in the health care system in New York undermined the ability of the state's prospective rate-setting system to control hospital costs for non-Medicare payers. The number of HMOs operating in New York more than doubled from 1984 to 1996. In 1984, thirteen HMOs enrolled roughly 1.3 million persons; a decade later, more than 4.3 million New Yorkers were enrolled in thirty HMOs, twelve prepaid health service plans, and sixteen partially capitated health plans (New York State 1995). The Pataki administration's task force on reforming the state's health care financing system argued that the rapid growth of managed care in New York State had made NYPHRM an anachronism (New York Department of Health 1995b). Critics alleged that hospital payment rates set by the state under NYPHRM were higher than the rates that payers could negotiate with institutions through volume discounts. In addition, NYPHRM's ability to control system-wide health care costs was limited, for an increasing proportion of patients were covered by managed care plans which were free to negotiate rates with providers, while a shrinking proportion of the population was enrolled in plans whose rates were set by the state. Furthermore, the task force concluded that since NYPHRM did not establish rates for outpatient services, its ability to control costs was increasingly limited. Finally, the unanimous report of the task force also indicted that the state's system of "targeted infusions" for charity care, capital projects, and medical education was inefficient and misdirected.[11]

Legal challenges to the constitutionality of the state's rate-setting methodology, and in particular to the legally mandated price differentials between charge payers (e.g., commercial insurers) and the rates paid by Blue Cross and Medicaid, also contributed to the demise of state regulation of health care financing. As one senior official in the state's Department of Health noted in 1990, "We're in court all the time, but generally we're sustained. We generally don't get challenged over the state's authority to set rates, but [rather] over their interpretation; providers are generally under the impression that the state has the statutory authority [to regulate payments to hospitals]." Hospitals in New York repeatedly challenged both the state's statutory authority and specific interpretations of rules and regulations that govern the payment system.

In a series of decisions, state courts had repeatedly upheld the scope of state regulatory powers over the industry during the 1970s and 1980s. In *Jewish Memorial Hospital v. Whalen*, the Court of Appeals upheld both the peer groupings established by the Cost Control Act (Chapter 957 of the Public Laws of 1969) and the Commissioner of Health's authority to retroactively lower previously established interim payment rates for inpatient hospital services. Similarly, the new regulatory powers conferred on the commissioner to close "unneeded" hospital facilities by the legislature (Chapter 76 of the New York Public Laws of 1976) were upheld by the Court of Appeals in *Hamptons Hospital and Medical Center v. Moore* in 1981. In its opinion, the court declared that "it requires no documentation to demonstrate the catastrophic economic consequences which might attend the construction of unneeded health care facilities."

The hospital industry has an uneven track record in its confrontations with the Department of Health, particularly where the department's rule-making authority is concerned. A new round of regulations promulgated in 1987, which amended the state's basic operating requirements for hospitals, prompted new charges of "micro-management" by the hospital industry and reflected a widely shared belief among providers that the Department of Health had once again overstepped the scope of legitimate authority. After the U.S. Health Care Financing Administration published the first major revision of its guidelines for participating hospitals in the Medicare and Medicaid programs, New York was required by statute to revise its own mini-mum standards of hospital operation, which are mandated to be at least as strict as their federal counterparts (New York Department of Health 1990b). The new regulations, known as Part 405, amended Article 28 of the state's public health law and mandated that hospitals provide a wider range of patient services and limited administrators' discretion on many routine issues of hospital management.[12]

New York's requirements far exceeded federal requirements for certification under the Medicare and Medicaid programs. Not surprisingly, the principal bone of contention boiled down to the cost of implementing the new measures; HANYS estimated the cost at more than $270 million. The Department of Health, in contrast, argued that the new requirements would cost no more than $55 million.[13] To cover Medicare's share of the new costs, the DOH decided not to adopt new regulations but rather adjusted the rates of all non-Medicare payers upward, effectively shifting the burden of costs from the public to the private sector. At this, Blue Cross sued on behalf of the state's private insurers, contending that the DOH could not force other payers to pick up Medicare's fiscal obligations for implementing the reforms contained in Part 405.

Soon after, the hospital association filed suit in the state Supreme Court, alleging that the state had overstepped its authority with the new regulations.[14] While HANYS' suit was dismissed as "speculative" and "political" in nature, the court found in favor of Blue Cross and ordered that Blue Cross rates had to be reduced to eliminate Medicare's share of the costs. The court's decision also ordered the hospitals, rather than the state, to reimburse Blue Cross for more than $55 million in payments received under the Department of Health's adjusted payment scheme. While this incident was only one in a series of heated conflicts, it illustrates the fundamental conflict of interest among the two most powerful private players in the reimbursement process. The acerbic relationship between Blue Cross and the hospital industry defines the process of interest group intermediation in the Empire State, for the discord among private interests greatly enhances the autonomy and discretion of state officials.

Most legal challenges to the payment system prior to 1993 focused upon fairly specific disagreements over the adequacy of reimburse-ment.[15] The basic legitimacy of the state's role in regulating reimbursement, maintaining a fixed differential among payers, and assessing surcharges on hospital care to finance various public policy goals were not in doubt following the Court of Appeals decision in *Rebaldo v. Cuomo* in 1984. Under these conditions, winning lawsuits against the state was difficult, for the exact definitions of "reasonable and adequate" rates and the determination of whether a hospital was operating "efficiently and effectively" were left to the discretion of the Commissioner of Health. New York's power to regulate the hospital industry faced its most serious challenge in 1993 when the Travelers Insurance Company challenged its establishment of differential reimbursement rates for commercial insurance companies on the grounds that state action was preempted by the federal Employee Retirement and Income Security Act (ERISA). NYPHRM IV required commercially insured patients to pay 13% more than the standard DRG rate for patients covered by Medicaid or Blue Cross; the extra billings were retained by the hospital providing services to offset losses from uncompensated care. In addition, commercially insured patients were required to pay an additional 11% surcharge, which was turned over to the state; in sum, rates of reimbursement for commercially insured patients exceeded the DRG rate by 24%.[16] Blue Cross and the Hospital Association of New York State (HANYS) joined the state as codefendants in the case in an effort to preserve the differential.

The fate of NYPHRM's rate-setting controls remained in doubt for more than a year. Both U.S. District Court Judge Louis Freeh and the Court of Appeals (2nd Circuit) declared that the legislatively mandated differential "regulated the terms of employee benefit plans" in violation of ERISA's preemption clause.[17] Although the state's power to regulate hospital rates for public policy purposes was later upheld on appeal to the U.S. Supreme Court, NYPHRM operated in a state of legal limbo for more than two years.[18] Continued uncertainty about the future of the state's health care financing system led legislators and industry groups to explore alternative options for controlling costs.

During the 1994 gubernatorial campaign, it became increasingly apparent that the principal alternative to state rate-setting was a dramatic increase in the number of New Yorkers enrolled in managed care plans. The election of George Pataki solidified the legitimacy of competitive options for reforming New York's health care system, for the new governor promised to harness the potential of managed care to control costs and improve the uneven quality of services provided to recipients. In addition, the Pataki administration ushered in a new philosophy of government. Soon after his inauguration, Pataki declared that "this government not only spends too much and taxes too much, it regulates too much" (Pataki 1995). The governor promised tax cuts and regulatory reform in an effort to stimulate job growth and stem the mass exodus of corporations from the state. Proposals for deregulating the hospital industry were welcomed by many local governments, whose share of state Medicaid costs had continued to rise under NYPHRM. In Albany and Rensselaer counties, for example, local Medicaid costs more than doubled from 1989 to 1993 (Picchi 1994). By 1995, the state's rate-setting system had many detractors and few supporters. In her final report to the governor, Health Commissioner Barbara DeBuono declared that the members of the task force on reforming NYPHRM had reached "unanimous agreement . . . that the current NYPHRM legislation does not meet the state's goals for health care in light of dramatic changes taking place in health care delivery through the emergence of managed care" (New York Department of Public Health 1995b).

Finally, leadership changes within the Department of Health contributed to a steady decline in its influence over health care policymaking. The loss of David Axelrod as Commissioner in 1991 was a devastating blow, for the Cuomo administration had exercised substantial deference to his policy agenda over the previous decade. Axelrod's charisma and defining presence left a gaping hole in the state's health care policy regime, for he was the most energetic and committed proponent of expanded state oversight over the hospital industry as a means of controlling costs and protecting patient rights. While fundamental changes were occurring in the health care system, the department operated with interim leadership for nearly two years until the appointment of Marc Chassin in 1992. In subsequent years, the department has suffered a "brain drain" from its senior leadership ranks, as experienced senior administrators such as Raymond Sweeney, the director of the Office of Health Systems Management since 1984, left state government. By the mid-1990s, the department presided over an unpopular reimbursement system which had little support from state legislators, industry groups, and the executive branch. The appointment of Barbara DeBuono as commissioner in 1995 exemplified the shift in the department's leadership priorities, for the new director was an ardent proponent of competition in the health sector.

Taken together, the sea change in health care financing in New York State is best explained by a confluence of forces. Shifting market conditions undermined business support for rate-setting and limited the ability of the state's prospective payment system to control system-wide costs. Legal challenges to NYPHRM in the mid-1990s also weakened policymakers' diffuse support for regulatory solutions to health care cost containment; continued uncertainty over the future of the payment system offered proponents of deregulation an opportunity to tout the potential of managed care to bring ballooning Medicaid costs under control. In the end, however, the impetus for changing New

York State's health care system came from within the state, as the governor's Ad Hoc Task Force on NYPHRM served as a policy incubator for deregulatory reform. In the end, the norms and principles which had sustained the imposition of regulatory controls over the health care industry for more than two decades fell out of favor.

New York State's health care financing regime presents a curious amalgam, for while the state Medicaid program continues to operate on a fee-for-service basis, third-party payers are free to negotiate their rates with health care providers. State officials in New York presided over the creation of an imposed regulatory regime in the early 1970s; continued fiscal stress and the burdens imposed by the state's liberal network of social programs helped to solidify the state's interest in health care cost containment during the 1980s. State autonomy, however, is not static. The transformation of New York State's imposed health policy regime underscores the tenuousness of state efforts to design and implement coercive policy choices over the objections of societal groups. Even where state regulatory programs are highly institutionalized, as in New York, underlying shifts in the political and economic climate can weaken support for the extension of public authority.

CHAPTER NOTES

1. Under NYPHRM III, payment to hospitals was based partially on their own costs and partially on the average cost for a peer group of hospitals: the pricing component's share of total hospital reimbursement, however, increased from 10% in 1988 to 55% in 1990.

2. The Department of Health used data provided by hospitals under the provisions of the Metcalf-McClosky Act to determine each institution's historical costs. Historical costs were adjusted each year for inflation after being subjected to "efficiency standards" that removed any expenses which were not reimbursable under the state's Medicaid formula. After this initial calculation, each hospital's ancillary costs and length of stay were compared to those of peer institutions: the average routine cost and ancillary cost per patient day were adjusted for differences in hospital case mix. Costs which exceeded the group average were disallowed. Once a hospital's costs were determined, they were divided by the institution's patient days in 1981 (the base year) to arrive at an operating per diem reimbursement rate. Capital costs were determined in a similar fashion, except that the utilization of services, rather than 1981 patient days, were used to compute the per diem rate. Significantly, capital costs were not adjusted for inflation.

3. Each hospital's reimbursement under the new program was based on the costs of a peer group of comparable hospitals. The actual rate of reimbursement was a blend of the hospital's own costs, or hospital-specific price, and the average costs of peer institutions, known as the group price.

4. For an excellent discussion of New York's bad debt and free care pools, see Thorpe and Spencer (1991).

5. New York's per diem rate-setting system was considerably more stringent than Medicare's new PPS. After adjusting for inflation, Medicare's costs for inpatient care using PPS in 1986 were $400 million more than under NYPHRM I's per diem methodology.

6. While NYPHRM III incorporated the existing Medicare DRG classification system, the state's Department of Health made several changes to accommodate the PPS categories to the peculiar circumstances of the Empire State. The initial version of NYPHRM III introduced new DRG categories for neonatal care and AIDS; subsequent revisions created 54 new DRGs to reflect major complications and comorbidities, thus increasing the system's ability to "account for differences in costs among patients and allowing payments for the specific DRGs to be more sensitive to the actual cost of treating these patients" (New York State Department of Health 1990b, 30). In addition, modifications to the payment system in 1990 introduced new classifications for high-risk obstetrical care, compulsive eating disorders, and orthopedic and spinal procedures; by 1995, the state's DRG system included more than 700 diagnostic categories.

7. The system established four separate reimbursement rates: Blue Cross and Medicaid reimburse providers on the same basis and provide the baseline for other payers' rate computations. Commercial insurers, the state worker's compensation fund, and no-fault insurance funds pay hospitals at the Blue Cross rate plus 13%, while self-paying patients may pay a maximum of the commercial insurers' DRG rate plus 20%. HMOs were treated separately under NYPHRM III as the only payers allowed to negotiate reimbursement rates directly with providers.

8. The pluralistic revenue stream of nonprofit hospitals is a by-product of their legal status. As nonprofit institutions with strong support in their local communities, voluntary hospitals benefit from fundraising drives, gifts, and other contributions that their for-profit competitors do not have access to. In addition, nonprofit institutions are often able to obtain financing at more favorable rates than other businesses.

9. In addition to their base salary, members receive a reimbursement of $89 per day to cover the cost of expenses while the legislature is in session; members may also qualify for additional benefits "in lieu of salary."

10. See Wilson's (1989) excellent discussion of the impact of beliefs and professional norms on organizational behavior in the U.S. Forest Service, the Federal Trade Commission, and other federal agencies. Since professional training in economics provides individuals with both analytical tools and a reference group of peers with a shared "world view" regarding industrial organization, it is not surprising that departmental policy was often closely based upon prevailing interpretations of the behavior of nonprofit institutions.

11. The task force argued that the existing system of state support for uncompensated care was "inappropriately targeted" on two counts. First, by failing to distinguish between charity care and "operating inefficiencies," the state effectively subsidized institutional operating budgets. In addition, since state funding for uncompensated care was targeted at inpatient, rather than

ambulatory settings, NYPHRM offered few incentives to develop community based primary care services to improve the health of indigent patients.

12. The Part 405 regulations required hospitals to hire translators to serve non-English-speaking patients and their families, encouraged the hiring and training of bilingual staff members, set limits on the number of hours interns could work, imposed new controls on prescription drug usage, and addressed a host of associated issues that had previously been decided by hospital administrators.

13. This figure did not represent the Department of Health's commitment of new resources, however, for the state's assessment of reimbursable expenses only totaled $44 million, of which $22 million represented Medicare's share. Hence, in the eyes of Commissioner David Axelrod, the state was only obliged to produce $22 million in additional revenues to implement the new regulations.

14. In New York the Supreme Court is actually the lowest level of the state court system, rather than a court of appeals.

15. Two court decisions from the past decade illustrate this point. While the New York State Supreme Court found that the Commissioner of Health (David Axelrod) could not require the state's Blue Cross and Blue Shield plans to reimburse hospitals for costs associated with treating Medicare patients in *New York State Conference of Blue Cross & Blue Shield Plans v. Axelrod* (1989), Judge Lawrence Kahn's opinion left the Department of Health's rule-making authority on hospital reimbursement issues untouched. In a related case in 1989 (*Hospital Association of New York State et. al v. Axelrod, Perales, and State Hospital Planning and Review Council*) the court rejected the hospital's contention that the department's stringent new minimum operating standards, expected to cost the industry millions of dollars statewide, were "arbitrary, capricious, and an abuse of discretion in that they require[d] employment of additional personnel in numbers which exceed the available labor supply to such an extent that compliance is impossible."

16. See the majority opinion in *N.Y. Conference of Blue Cross and Blue Shield Plans v. Travelers Insurance* (1995, 1674).

17. The District Court overturned the NYPHRM regulations in the case of *Travelers Insurance Co. v. Cuomo.* The preemption clause has been a bane for state health reform efforts in every state except Hawaii, which obtained a congressional exemption from ERISA for its universal health insurance program using an employer mandate in 1975. Under section 514 (a), ERISA "shall supersede any and all state laws insofar as they . . . relate to any employee benefit plan" (*N.Y. Conference of Blue Cross and Blue Shield Plans v. Travelers Insurance* 1995, 1675). For a more extensive discussion of ERISA's impact on state health reform efforts, see Chirba-Martin and Brennan (1994).

18. Since NYPHRM's differentials "affect only indirectly the relative prices of insurance policies, a result no different from myriad state laws in areas traditionally subject to local regulation," the court upheld the state's power to set rates and establish differentials among third-party payers, effectively ending further challenges to the legitimacy of New York's hospital cost-containment efforts.

4

Massachusetts: Competition and Consensus in a Negotiated Policy Regime

> "We've got to hold the hospitals back from the gorging they've been doing ... it's an orgy," Nelson Gifford, Chairman of the Massachusetts Business Roundtable, 1987.

> "You don't have to be a brain surgeon to see if we can't bring the [Medicaid] program under control it is going to eat the rest of state government alive," Charles Baker, Jr., Secretary of Health and Human Services, 1993.

Hospital cost containment in Massachusetts has been governed by a negotiated policy regime over the past two decades. Public officials in the Bay State have supported policies to promote competition among hospitals since the late 1970s. In the early 1980s, state officials sought to foster competition through a progressive all-payer rate-setting methodology. Massachusetts' rate-setting system was hammered out through a process of meso-corporatist bargaining in the early 1980s (Bergthold 1988) and enjoyed strong support from business groups and health insurers through the mid-1980s. After 1990, however, state officials abandoned their previous efforts to force hospitals to compete through rate-setting. Changes in the state's health insurance marketplace and growing competition among hospitals for a declining pool of paying patients led the state to embrace a "prudent purchasing" policy toward cost containment. Although the state no longer set prices for hospital reimbursement, public officials retained a significant role in expanding care for the uninsured, financing uncompensated care, and monitoring the quality of health care services in the increasingly competitive health care marketplace in Massachusetts.

Public officials in Massachusetts have consistently articulated the state's interest in controlling costs in negotiations with providers, third-party payers, and representatives from the business community. The state, however, has found it difficult to implement restrictive cost-containment initiatives in the face of societal opposition. Successful efforts to control costs have enjoyed broad-based support from the private sector. Since health care policy-making is a high-visibility issue in the Bay State, conflict among providers and payers has been commonplace. Until the 1990s, most conflicts centered around technical issues related to the adequacy of reimbursement, financing uncompensated care, assisting certain hospitals that had been penalized by the reimbursement methodology, and the most effective means to control costs without unduly penalizing providers. Relationships among the principal actors in the state's health policy regime deteriorated swiftly after the passage of the Dukakis administration's universal health care plan in 1988. As the state's economy fell into a tailspin, spiraling Medicaid costs prompted state officials to slow payments to providers, reduce funding for uncompensated care, and postpone plans to expand insurance to the working poor and uninsured. In the face of a growing fiscal crisis, Massachusetts' rate-setting system lost support from payers and providers alike. The election of Governor William Weld, a staunch fiscal conservative who championed deregulation and competition throughout the 1990 gubernatorial campaign, signaled the end of an era for hospital cost containment in the Bay State; by the end of 1991, legislators approved a sweeping plan to deregulate the state's health care financing system, effectively gutting the universal health care act passed three years before.

The state returned to a position of national policy leadership in the mid-1990s by aggressively moving Medicaid beneficiaries into managed care. The size and economic importance of the health care industry in Massachusetts limits the ability of state officials to impose restrictive payment policies on providers without strong support from societal groups. Massachusetts' decision to deregulate hospital payment, however, did not signal a wholesale withdrawal of state intervention in health care policy-making. Policymakers remain committed to expanding access to health care, fostering competition, and mediating the impact of managed care on patients and physicians. Tensions over financing uncompensated care and the introduction of for-profit hospital chains have strained relationships among providers, payers, and the state in recent years.

THE POLICY-MAKING ENVIRONMENT IN MASSACHUSETTS

Health care policy-making is a high-profile issue in Massachusetts and regularly occupies center stage in legislative debates. Many of the nation's premier teaching hospitals and research institutions are located in the greater Boston area; health care is one of the largest and fastest growing areas of the Massachusetts economy. In 1995, three hospitals (Beth Israel, Brigham and Women's, and Massachusetts General Hospital) and two health plans (Blue Cross and Harvard Community Health Plan) were among the twenty-five largest employers in the state. Overall, the health care industry is the second largest employer in Massachusetts, employing more than 310,000 workers in 1995 (10.5% of the state's work force). The extraordinary concentration of health care facilities and personnel, however, has also contributed to the high cost of health care in Massachusetts. In response to growing competition among providers, the pace of vertical and horizontal merger activity increased dramatically after 1991.

As one of the state's largest employers, hospitals have a strong political presence; the Massachusetts Hospital Association (MHA) actively lobbies legislators, state agencies, and the governor's office on matters that affect its membership. In addition to its own staff of paid lobbyists, however, the MHA also seeks to mobilize grass-roots support for policies that benefit the hospital industry by encouraging representatives from its member institutions to contact their local legislative delegations. Indeed, hospitals were frequently mentioned by legislators and their staffs as one of the most active lobbying groups in the state (Berg 1993). Hospitals acceded to the creation of the state's all-payer rate-setting system in the early 1980s, but the industry won significant financial concessions from state legislators in exchange for its support for universal health insurance in 1988.

Unfortunately for the MHA and its members, an unprecedented fiscal crisis led the Dukakis administration to curtail, not expand, payments to providers and postpone or scale back state efforts to subsidize care for the uninsured as the 1980s drew to a close. In 1989, the MHA sued the Department of Public Welfare over a growing backlog of unpaid Medicaid bills. Industry representatives charged that the department "created a seemingly endless maze of obstacles for not paying its bills" in an effort to balance the state budget (quoted in Loth 1989). By 1989, the state owed providers more than $670 million in overdue Medicaid payments, including more than $200 million in unpaid rate increases approved in 1985 and 1986. Legislators avoided a protracted legal battle with the hospital industry by approving the sale of bonds to finance $488 million in past-due payments (Wallin 1995, 255). In the years following the state's recovery from the fiscal crisis of 1989–91, the industry's financial health and its relationship with state officials improved. In 1996, approximately three out of four hospitals in the state reported an operating surplus, although profit margins remained thin (Stein 1996a). Growing competition, however, forced many of the state's largest teaching hospitals to lay off workers and consolidate operations in an effort to cut costs.

The hospital industry in Massachusetts was transformed by a series of high profile mergers and acquisitions during the 1990s.[1] In 1996, for-profit hospital chains made their first significant inroads in the state's health care market, as OrNda Corp. purchased St. Vincent's Hospital in Worcester and Columbia/HCA acquired a controlling interest in MetroWest Medical Center in Framingham (Pham 1996b). After 1993, the pace of consolidation among hospitals transformed the state's health care system, particularly in the greater Boston area. The list of mergers included some of the state's largest and most respected institutions; after Brigham and Women's Hospital joined Massachusetts General Hospital to form Partners Health Care System, Beth Israel Hospital merged with Deaconess Hospital to form Care Group and New England Medical Center was acquired by Lifespan, a nonprofit hospital chain based in Rhode Island. In one of the state's most controversial mergers, Boston University Medical Center merged with Boston City Hospital in 1996, setting off a round of layoffs and cost-cutting moves.[2] From 1992 to 1994, more than one in five hospitals in Massachusetts were involved in mergers, acquisitions, or contractual affiliations with other institutions or corporations (Hegarty 1994).

Relations between hospitals, health insurers, and the business community have soured in recent years as the state's health care industry lurched toward competition. Business groups, whose support was instrumental in creating the state's all-payer rate-setting system in the 1980s, strongly opposed any additional taxes to fund uncompensated care as an unacceptable burden on employers (Stein 1990a). Insurers, for their part, became increasingly aggressive in price negotiations with hospitals following the deregulation of the Massachusetts hospital rate-setting system in 1991. During the debate over renewing the state's hospital financing system in 1991, MHA president Steven Hegarty warned that "Blue Cross is so big that they may be able to reshape the entire system. They may decide who lives and who dies in the hospital world" (quoted in Stein 1991a). Five years later, Hegarty's warning appeared prescient, as Blue Cross terminated its contracts with hospitals that refused to accede to the company's demands for price concessions (Knox 1996b).

Health insurers welcomed the growth of market competition in the Massachusetts health care industry. With the highest managed care market penetration of any state in the nation, Massachusetts offered an intensely competitive environment for third-party payers. In 1993, 38.9% of the state's population were enrolled in HMOs (Marion Merrill

Dow 1994). Consolidation has also reshaped the face of the health insurance industry in Massachusetts, as two of the state's largest HMOs (Harvard Community Health Plan and Pilgrim Health Care) merged in 1995; the new company, Harvard Pilgrim Health Care, is now the largest HMO in New England with more than 1.1 million members (Pham 1996a). Since Massachusetts residents may choose from more than fifteen separate managed care organizations, businesses have aggressively sought to wring price concessions from HMOs (Stein 1996c). In particular, the Massachusetts Healthcare Purchaser Group (MHPG), representing several of the state's largest employers, has challenged payers to either hold the line on premium increases or cut their rates for each year since 1993. In a startling development, the average monthly HMO premium in Massachusetts fell from $156 per subscriber in 1995 to $147 in 1996 (Pham 1996c). Insurers demanded steep discounts from providers in exchange for guaranteed patient volume. In the words of one Blue Cross executive, "We are saying to the hospitals, 'Unless you can be more reasonable, we can't use you. . . . We can walk away'" (quoted in Stein 1991b, 30).

Blue Cross and Blue Shield of Massachusetts has been one of the most powerful advocates for reforming the state's hospital financing system over the past decade. The company's premiums rose considerably during the 1980s, but the regulated reimbursement system established in the 1970s limited its ability to bargain for discounted rates with providers. Facing massive losses by the end of the 1980s, Blue Cross welcomed the opportunity to use its purchasing power to negotiate volume discounts with providers. By 1991, Blue Cross and Blue Shield of Massachusetts had been targeted as one of the nation's most financially troubled Blue Cross plans (Pulliam 1991; U.S. General Accounting Office 1994).

The company's managerial difficulties are legendary in Massachusetts. After investing more than $80 million in a new computer system to process claims, Blue Cross pulled the plug on the project after auditors warned that its "System 21" was an expensive failure (Stein 1991b; Edelman 1991). To make matters worse, rapidly rising cost and administrative inefficiency led to the loss of the company's most lucrative group contract, as the commonwealth refused to renew its standard health insurance package for state employees in 1990. The Weld administration's plan for hospital reform offered Blue Cross and all other insurers (including Medicaid) the opportunity to selectively contract with hospitals. After earning modest profits in the early 1990s, Blue Cross reported losses of more than $70 million in 1996, prompting company officials to seek state assistance to subsidize the cost of offering traditional indemnity coverage (Pham 1996d).

Businesses first entered health care financing debates during the early 1980s in response to a threat by the state's largest commercial insurers to pull out of the Bay State's insurance market (Bergthold 1988). Commercial insurers were losing money at an unprecedented rate as a result of the high cost of health care in Massachusetts and the rising differential between their rates and those of Blue Cross, which were capped under the existing reimbursement system. The Massachusetts Business Roundtable (MBRT) and the Associated Industries of Massachusetts (AIM) led the coalition pressing for an all-payer rate-setting system in order to preserve choice among insurance options for Bay State businesses. Businesses supported the state's all-payer rate-setting methodology as a means of controlling costs and limiting cost shifting among payers through the mid-1980s (Bergthold 1990b). Legislative bargaining over the renewal of the hospital reimbursement system in 1988, however, soon became enmeshed in the emerging debate over health care reform. As the principal focus of negotiations over a new payment system shifted from cost containment to universal health insurance, businesses grew increasingly disillusioned with state-sponsored solutions to control their health care costs (Bergthold 1990a).

Legislators sweetened the fiscal incentives for providers in order to win hospitals' support for universal health insurance, significantly weakening the principal cost-containment provisions of the state's rate-setting system in the process. The passage of Chapter 23 of the Massachusetts Public Laws of 1988 left business leaders with a profound sense of disillusionment over legislative solutions to control health care costs. In addition, leadership changes at the MBRT prompted business groups to turn their attention away from health care reform to issues such as tax reform and economic development after 1988. In the 1990s, business groups increasingly sought to control health care costs through private, not public, initiatives. On the one hand, Digital Equipment Corporation and other major employers have provided strong financial incentives for their employees to enroll in high-quality HMOs which meet the company's stringent performance standards (Digital Equipment Corporation 1995). In Digital's case, benefits managers did not eliminate choice of health insurance options, but instead linked the company's contribution to the benchmark price of the lowest-cost managed care organization that met its performance standards. The company's cost was the same regardless of the insurance option selected by employees, who were responsible for the difference in cost between the lowest-cost plan and their own.[3]

In addition to more aggressive benefits management strategies, however, employers in Massachusetts sought to increase their leverage over providers and health insurers by forming the Massachusetts Healthcare Purchaser Group in 1992. The new organization, representing nearly a million subscribers, released annual "report cards" on the quality and value of the state's major managed care plans and challenged insurers to hold price increases to a predetermined ceiling (Wise 1994). MHPG's report cards, however, generated considerable controversy. In 1996, Blue Cross and Blue Shield of Massachusetts indicated that it would no longer participate in the annual evaluation after its HMO Blue plan received poor ratings in patient satisfaction.

In the face of stable, or declining, health insurance premiums for employees enrolled in managed care plans, health care costs were no longer viewed in crisis terms by business organizations in the mid-1990s. Business leaders, however, remained wary of state proposals to expand health insurance coverage to the uninsured. At the request of the Weld administration, legislators repealed the unimplemented "pay or play" employer mandate in 1996. Nevertheless, legislative supporters continued to press for legislation which would require all businesses in the state to offer coverage to their employees or pay $1,200 per employee to the state. Although business leaders acknowledged that "the issue of the uninsured is a major question," the AIM joined small businesses in condemning the proposal, citing concerns about "one state doing it on its own" (quoted in Knox 1996a). In short, while businesses have not disengaged themselves from health care policy-making, they no longer look to the state for solutions to controlling their health care costs.

Over the past decade, the growing interest of business groups in health care policy-making was paralleled by the emergence of strong public interest groups advocating for consumers, the elderly, the disabled, and the uninsured. In the mid-1980s, the lobbying efforts of Health Care for All, a grass-roots advocacy group committed to expanding access to health insurance, helped to define the legislative agenda for reforming the state's health care financing system (Goldberger 1990). Health Care for All lobbied heavily for the passage of the Dukakis administration's Health Security Act in 1988 and vigorously opposed efforts to postpone or repeal its provisions in the early 1990s. In recent years, the organization has pressed for reforms to the state's uncompensated care fund and campaigned for strict state oversight of for-profit hospital mergers. In 1996, the advocacy group's newly formed legal arm, Health Law Associates, successfully negotiated agreements with the Department of Public Health to maintain access to emergency services and walk-in clinics for residents of Worcester County after the closure of a local hospital (McNamara 1996). Although Health Care for All has not been a regular participant in the quasi-corporatist bargaining which shaped health care policy in Massachusetts, it remains a vocal advocate for consumers and the poor in legislative debates.

HEALTH CARE COST CONTAINMENT IN MASSACHUSETTS

Massachusetts' early efforts to control hospital costs did not seriously threaten the fiscal health or managerial autonomy of health care providers. State intervention in the hospital reimbursement process began in 1968 when the legislature established the Massachusetts Rate-Setting Commission (MRSC) and granted it the authority to determine "fair and reasonable" rates of reimbursement for health care services; capital expenditure review, known as "determination of need" in Massachusetts, followed in 1971. Prior to 1975, the system was entirely retrospective in nature, for payment to providers was determined by computing the ratio of costs to billed charges. Interim rates were set by the MRSC, using hospitals' unaudited cost and charge data. Under this methodology, final payment rates could not be computed until the data was audited and "excessive" charges or uncovered services were disallowed. A year or more typically passed before a reaching a final settlement that determined whether the interim rates had underpaid or overpaid providers (Sahlein 1973). In addition,

> since the laws governing the establishment of rates provide no specific guidance as to what constitutes a reasonable cost, Commission auditors are severely limited in their ability to disallow expenditures. Thus, almost all expenditures are accepted as reimbursable. This leaves hospitals free to budget for any expenditure levels deemed appropriate, knowing that the portion for publicly aided patients can be billed in full to the commonwealth (Sahlein 1973, 3).

By 1975, however, the state's ballooning $500 million budget deficit prompted the Dukakis administration to search for a more effective means of controlling Medicaid costs (Kronick 1990). The passage of Chapter 409 in 1976 gave state policymakers additional leverage over total hospital spending in the commonwealth by granting the MRSC the authority to set and review rates for Blue Cross, Medicaid, and charge-based payers. Beginning in 1976, the MRSC used different reimbursement methodologies to set rates for Medicaid, private insurers, and Blue Cross.[4] Hospitals were required to submit estimates of past, present, and current year costs to the MRSC, which then determined each institution's "reasonable financial requirements." With these financial requirements in hand, the MRSC established a charge structure to enable hospitals to meet their general operating costs, plus the cost of expected changes in volume and the provision of new services, and maintain funds for working capital (Esposito et al. 1982). The end result of using three very different methods for paying providers was a situation perfectly tailored for extensive cost shifting in which both Blue Cross and the commercial charge payers were saddled with higher rates. Continued cost shifting, in turn, led to a growing gap between Blue Cross premiums and those of commercial insurers.

Five years after its passage, the reimbursement system created by Chapter 409 was unstable.[5] In 1980, the MRSC had taken the unprecedented step of rejecting Blue Cross' master contract with the state's hospitals (HA-28) in an effort to prod providers to become more efficient. The MRSC's chairman, Steven Weiner, argued that the retrospective agreement proposed by Blue Cross was too lenient and pressed for the development of an all-payer rate-setting system (Bergthold 1988). Other events in 1980 also indicated that the tide was turning against the state's hospitals. The legislature's passage of a bill to cap the allowable increase in hospital charges to 11.5% over the previous year's level (Chapter 540) was a forerunner of things to come, for in 1981 the legislature approved a measure (Chapter 432) which limited the growth in hospitals' charges to the rate of inflation minus a 1.5% "productivity factor." The most significant modification of the Chapter 409 reimbursement system came in October 1981, however, when the MRSC approved a new contract (HA-29) between the hospitals and Blue Cross that radically altered the prevailing mode of provider reimbursement in the Bay State.

Under HA-29, Blue Cross shifted from a retrospective reimbursement methodology to a prospective one in which rates were determined by inflating costs in a base year (1981) to the rate year, after allowing for changes in volume and capital costs. Hospital revenues were based by computing a "maximum allowable cost" (MAC) for each institution.[6] If a hospital's actual costs exceeded the prenegotiated MAC, it absorbed the loss. Conversely, if costs fell below the MAC, the hospital was permitted to retain the difference, providing a strong incentive for institutions to improve the efficiency of their operations. Since the base year for computing hospital revenues did not change under HA-29 or its successor agreements in the 1980s, however, institutions that had lower costs in FY1981 were actually penalized by the new reimbursement system.

The passage of Chapter 372 in 1982 extended the principles of HA-29 to all payers in the commonwealth by adopting an all-payer rate-setting system. The new reimbursement methodology encouraged hospitals to reduce the use of inpatient services by shifting patient care to less expensive outpatient settings and promised to reimburse hospitals for the cost of bad debts and charity care. Revenue compliance under the new system was based on hospitals' gross patient service revenues (GPSR), or total charges from all payers. The all-payer system also expanded the "productivity" incentives introduced in 1981; under Chapter 372 the budgeted cost base used to compute hospitals' reimbursement under both Medicare and Medicaid was reduced by 2% in 1983 and 1984. As Blue Cross noted in an internal memorandum evaluating the all-payer system, this permanently reduced hospitals' revenues, for the "productivity requirements are recurring and cumulative."

Massachusetts' all-payer system operated under a waiver from HCFA from 1983–1985, when Medicare withdrew in favor of its new prospective payment system. Medicare's withdrawal necessitated two significant changes in the state's reimbursement methodology. Medicare's use of a DRG-based payment system meant that its payments to hospitals were no longer related to their actual charges; other insurers sought to protect themselves from excessive cost-shifting behavior by hospitals. The passage of Chapter 574 in 1985 was intended to control the ability of hospitals to shift costs for both inpatient and outpatient services. After 1985, hospitals' compliance with the system's cost-control goals was based upon institutions' allowed non-Medicare gross patient service revenues (NMGPSR) rather than their total charges (GPSR). The new Blue Cross master contract authorized by Chapter 574 (HA-30) also extended the 2% productivity requirement introduced in 1982 to all payers. In addition, Chapter 574 reallocated the costs of free care and bad debts previously borne by Medicare to the remaining payers in the system.

After the expiration of Chapter 574 in 1988, hospitals pressed for changes in the state's reimbursement methodology to ease the stress on hospitals that experienced a decline in patient volume and to compensate "low base cost" hospitals that had been penalized for their efficiency in FY1981. In exchange for their support of the Dukakis administration's universal health care proposals, hospitals exacted promises from the state to (1) provide compensation for reduced Medicare reimbursements, losses due to Medicare's prospective payment system, (2) minimize providers' liability for "uncompensated care" by expanding health insurance coverage to all residents, and (3) increase state funding for bad debt and free care. Although the new reimbursement methodology created by Chapter 23 retained the MAC-based system introduced 1982, it abandoned the productivity factors that had provided hospitals with a powerful fiscal incentive to cut costs since 1981. In addition, the 1988 legislation added a special fund to provide for pay raises above the salary cap, contributing to the inflationary wage spiral caused by a regional shortage of nurses and other allied health professionals.

The emerging fiscal crisis in Massachusetts during 1989 and 1990 led to the postponement, and ultimate repeal, of many of the provisions contained in the Health Security Act. In particular, state funding for bad debt and charity care failed to reach promised levels, and without a waiver from the federal government, the proposed "pay or play" system of employer mandated health insurance was never implemented. By 1990, the existing reimbursement methodology satisfied none of the key participants in Massachusetts' health policy regime. Hospitals did not fully reap the benefits promised to them under Chapter 23, but feared the consequences of a deregulated marketplace. In contrast, Blue Cross and other third-party payers longed for an opportunity to use their market position to extract substantial discounts in negotiations with hospitals.

After a decade of establishing fixed differentials among payers, setting limits on gross hospital revenues and volume statistics, and approving exceptions to prospectively determined hospital budgets, the legislature ended the state's role in setting rates for non-Medicaid payers on December 31, 1991. The withdrawal of state oversight of health care financing was striking, for the legislation declared that "all purchasers and third party payers may enter into contractual arrangements with acute care hospitals for services. No such arrangement . . . shall be subject to prior approval by any public agency. . . ." In another significant departure, Chapter 495 also ended the state's commitment to reimbursing hospitals for the cost of bad debts; in a competitive health care system, institutions were expected to increase the vigilance of their collection efforts.

The deregulation of hospital rates, however, was only one component of the Weld administration's strategy to control runaway Medicaid costs. Mandatory enrollment of Medicaid beneficiaries in managed care represented the second element of the administration's cost-containment strategy. Beginning in January 1992, Massachusetts began enrolling all AFDC-eligible recipients in a comprehensive managed care program which assigned patients a primary care clinician and paid providers on a capitated basis for mental health and substance abuse services under a Freedom of Choice (Section 1915b) waiver from HCFA. By 1994, nearly 470,000 recipients were enrolled in the program, known as MassHealth (Commonwealth of Massachusetts 1994). Building upon its successful implementation of the primary care clinician program, Massachusetts successfully applied for a Section 1115 waiver to expand insurance coverage to the uninsured and strengthen the private health insurance market. In particular, the program targeted low-income workers, children, and families; the disabled; and persons unable to purchase private insurance due to pre-existing conditions and waiting periods (HCFA 1996a).

The state's managed care initiative represented a new approach to promoting competition in the health care marketplace. As the state noted in its 1994 waiver application, "Massachusetts has rejected the notion that improved access and effective cost-containment can be achieved through a large-scale expansion of the traditional Medicaid program. . . . Instead, Massachusetts' proposal seeks to expand insurance coverage through the use of market-based incentives for employers, employees, and insurance providers" (Commonwealth of Massachusetts 1994, 8–9). The Weld administration initially sought to fund the expanded coverage by tapping the revenues generated by the state's Uncompensated Care Pool; the legislature rejected the governor's plan in favor of an increase in the excise tax on tobacco products (Kong 1995; McDonough, Hager, and Rosman 1996).

Recent surveys of Medicaid beneficiaries conducted by the Division of Medical Assistance confirm that the state's managed care experiment has won over enrollees, as 91% of MassHealth members reported that they were satisfied with their overall access to care and 94% expressed satisfaction with the quality of services they received in 1995. Independent analyses of the state's managed care initiatives conducted by researchers at the University of Massachusetts-Boston concluded that the Medicaid's Primary Care Clinician Program (PCCP) saved nearly $20 million on primary care during the first year of the state's Section 1915 waiver (Stein 1994). After years of double-digit increases in Medicaid costs, the Weld administration's policy of negotiating steep discounts with providers resulted in substantial cost savings, as costs per beneficiary rose only 2% during FY1994. During FY1996, costs were projected to rise by 2.4%.

In the early 1980s, Massachusetts' all-payer rate-setting system won accolades for dramatically slowing the rate of hospital inflation and minimizing the ability of institutions to shift costs to other payers. The volume incentives and productivity factors that were first introduced in 1982 provided hospitals with a clear incentive to reduce their operating expenses and to limit the intensity of services provided to patients. Hospital inflation in Massachusetts was lower than both state and regional averages after the implementation of the state's prospective budgeting system. Total expenditures by community hospitals rose by 56.6% from 1981 to 1987; hospital expenditures in New England and the U.S. rose by 63.5% and 69.4%, respectively, during the same period. The cost-containment record of Massachusetts' all-payer rate-setting system also compared favorably with those in other rate-setting states prior to the passage of the state's universal health care plan in 1988. From 1981 to 1987, total hospital costs in Massachusetts also increased at a lower rate than in Maryland, New Jersey, and New York.

By 1986, hospitals were in better fiscal health than they had been before the expansion of the state's rate-setting controls. Before the introduction of the all-payer system, 66% of the state's hospitals reported operating surpluses; after five years of rate-setting, 77% of the state's hospitals were in the black (Knox 1987c). As the director of the MRSC's hospital bureau observed, "Despite a drop in hospital utilization there has not been a more marked deterioration in [hospitals'] fiscal health because they were able to raise unit charges. This is not, in our opinion, the hallmark of an industry showing great signs of price competitiveness" (quoted in Knox 1987c). In addition, the average age of hospitals' physical plants dropped 30% from 1984 to 1989, following more than $2.5 billion of new capital spending (Knox 1991c). By 1990, Massachusetts hospitals had the youngest physical plants in the Northeast. In the wake of the state's construction boom in the late 1980s, the average age of hospital facilities fell considerably below the regional and national averages (Cleverly 1993). As one former director of the MRSC's hospital bureau remarked, "Chapter 23 and Chapter 372 contained the same incentives, but the problem with Chapter 23 is that it just handed money over. Chapter 23 said that 'over the past six years we've done some things that weren't right, so in order to fix it we're going to pump some more money into the system.' The result was an 11% jump in one year and a huge increase in the base."

Few cases demonstrated the demise of cost containment as a priority for the state's hospital financing system more than the treatment of several "low base cost hospitals" under Chapter 23. One of the goals of the 1988 legislation was to redress the grievances of many hospitals that felt that they had been unfairly treated under the provisions of Chapters 372 and 574. The low base cost hospitals contended that they were penalized for their efficiency because they started out with a smaller base; since the MAC was a formula-driven process driven by institutions' costs in the base year, low base cost hospitals' revenues grew at a slower pace than those of "less efficient" institutions. As one MRSC commissioner recalled, "It wasn't a particularly analytic process for determining who were low base cost hospitals and what they would get. There wasn't an appropriate case mix adjustment for them, so that hospitals were considered [to have] low base costs simply because they had lower costs per discharge, [regardless of] whether they didn't take care of very complicated patients." In addition, some observers argued that the adjustment for low base cost hospitals was merely a high-tech version of pork barrel politics. As one Blue Cross executive quipped,

"Whidden Hospital gets a special low base cost adjustment; it's bundled together with other hospitals which had low CMADs. It's in Everett. So's the Speaker [George Kevarian]. You figure it out."

Adjustments for low base cost hospitals were not the only inflationary provisions hidden in the 1988 legislation: HA-31 also offered hospitals an opportunity to "rebase" their volume statistics.[7] The Bay State's universal health care law also promised to compensate hospitals for the fiscal burden imposed by Medicare's new prospective payment system by establishing a Medicare shortfall assistance fund. The actual disbursement of funds was left in the hands of the Massachusetts Hospital Association, although the distribution of uncompensated care funds was subject to review by the MRSC. However, as the chair of the MRSC argued, although "the Commission had to decide whether or not to accept it [the MHA's proposed distribution], we considered that if they had already weighed and balanced [the issues] among their membership and made tradeoffs, we would accept that unless it was inappropriate." The cumulative effect of these changes was staggering; the increase in the state's contribution to the free care and bad debt pools alone added $325 million to the hospitals' coffers in the first year of HA-31.

Contrary to hospitals' initial fears, the 1990s did not bring a rash of hospital closures despite growing competition in the state's health care marketplace. Although three acute-care hospitals closed their doors in the first three years after the end of state rate-setting controls on January 1, 1992, 15 other acute-care facilities were converted to other uses or permanently closed between 1985 and 1991 (Sessler 1994). Furthermore, Boston area teaching hospitals found themselves under attack in 1993 after a study by Nancy Kane, a professor at Harvard University's School of Public Health, revealed that the city's teaching hospitals retained more than $1.1 billion in discretionary cash (Knox 1993b).

By the mid-1990s, the consequences of Massachusetts' decision to deregulate hospital rates had confounded critics who had predicted rampant price inflation in the absence of regulatory controls over hospital revenues. By 1996, KPMG Peat Marwick reported that Massachusetts hospitals ranked seventh in the nation in cost effectiveness; hospital costs increased less than 2% in each of the preceding years and were nearly 11% below the national average after adjusting for differences in cost of living and case mix severity (KPMG Peat Marwick 1996). Intensified competition among hospitals for patient volume provided payers with unprecedented market leverage. In an effort to restore its waning fiscal health, Blue Cross demanded, and subsequently received, price discounts of 30% or more from its participating hospitals in eastern Massachusetts. Although Blue Cross was expected to save more

than $200 million annually from the move, the company's tough negoti-
ating posture exacerbated fiscal pressures on hospitals, who depended
on Blue Cross for approximately 20% of their patient revenues
(Knox 1996b).

THE NATURE OF THE DECISION-MAKING PROCESS

The vital importance of the hospital industry to the Bay State's economy
has limited the ability of public officials to impose regulatory solutions
upon hospitals without support from businesses and third-party payers. During the 1970s and 1980s, state officials formed partnerships with
key societal interests to design and implement new cost-containment
initiatives. Business groups joined hospitals, third-party payers, and
state officials to create Massachusetts' all-payer rate-setting system in
1982 and presided over a fragile coalition that negotiated successive
agreements in 1985 and 1988. Since policy was shaped through private
negotiations among state officials and powerful peak associations
which were then ratified by the legislature, Linda Bergthold (1988)
described health care policy-making in Massachusetts as a contemporary example of meso-corporatist bargaining. The corporatist moment
in Massachusetts, however, proved to be fleeting. The consensus over
health policy goals needed to sustain the expansion of state authority
over the hospital industry evaporated after 1988. Soon after, the uneasy
collaboration among businesses, hospitals, state officials, and third-
party payers collapsed in the face of an emerging fiscal crisis.

Negotiated regimes are characterized by recurring tensions among
public and private participants over the design and implementation
of state policies to control health care costs. The evolution of health
care policy in Massachusetts over the past two decades was shaped
by recurring fiscal crises, the incorporation of new groups into the
decision-making process, and the shifting policy image of health care
reform. State responses to fiscal crises in the 1970s and 1980s rejected
direct confrontation with health care providers in favor of "administrative" solutions; Medicaid reimbursement to providers continued to
increase during the recessions of 1974–75, 1981–82, and 1989–91. Early
in the decade, decision-making on health care financing was conducted
in private with little legislative debate and public participation; by
1987, health care policy-making resembled a pluralist free-for-all, as
new groups besieged the legislature in pursuit of new benefits or regulatory relief. Finally, the policy image of health care financing issues
shifted during the 1980s from an emphasis on cost control to expanding
access to care for the uninsured. Both public officials and private groups
have expressed support for policies designed to promote competition

in the health care system for more than a decade. Although businesses, payers, and providers continue to acknowledge the legitimacy of the state's role in health care financing, they no longer turn to the state to bring health care costs under control.

The evolution of health care policy-making in Massachusetts has been shaped by successive fiscal crises. Although fiscal crises led state officials to experiment with new approaches to hospital reimbursement, the health care industry in Massachusetts did not endure serious financial hardship as a result of the state's troubles. Instead, public officials adopted an accommodating stance towards the industry in each era. The state's first serious effort to regulate the hospital industry, in 1976, strengthened the MRSC's power to review hospital payment rates, but neither Governor Michael Dukakis nor the legislature sought draconian cuts in Medicaid reimbursement to erase the deficit, but rather resorted to a $450 million bond issue, cuts in welfare eligibility and benefits, and a $350 million tax increase to balance the budget (Peirce 1976). State officials also ratified the Reagan administration's budget cuts in Medicaid and AFDC after 1981; while payments to providers increased from 1982 to 1983, the caseloads for both programs declined by more than 20% during the same period (Howitt and Leftwich 1987).

Efforts to reform health care financing in Massachusetts since the late 1980s have been driven by the enormous fiscal burden imposed by the state Medicaid program. As state Representative Richard Voke, the chairman of the Massachusetts House Ways and Means Committee, argued, "Health care is frankly where it's all at. . . . We're not going to get this state on a sound fiscal basis unless and until major changes are made in that area" (quoted in Loth 1990a). Spiraling Medicaid costs exceeded the growth in overall state spending by a factor of five in the late 1980s and early 1990s, prompting both public and private decision makers to label the program as the state's principal "budget buster." As the House Ways and Means Committee concluded in 1990, "Health care costs are controlling state government, to the detriment of all other vital state systems" (Knox 1990a). From FY1988 to 1990, Medicaid costs rose an average of 19.4% a year.

The state's budgetary problems continued to deteriorate during the Dukakis administration's last year in office; by the end of 1990, Massachusetts faced a deficit of more than $1.2 billion. Layoffs, employee furloughs, and a near total shutdown of all nonessential state government services cast a pall over legislative debates on resolving the state's fiscal crisis. Massachusetts' fiscal woes were exacerbated by an ongoing controversy over the state's share of the Medicare shortfall assistance fund and free care/bad debt pools. In the face of a growing deficit, the Dukakis administration backed away from its earlier commitment to fully fund the programs created by the 1988 universal health care legislation. Upon learning of the administration's decision to withhold more than $200 million in 1989, Massachusetts Hospital Association (MHA) president Stephen Hegarty declared that "the entire hospital community shares a sense of betrayal given that . . . the governor's legislation would not have become law without the intense grassroots support of every hospital throughout the state" (quoted in Loth 1989). The industry's indignation was backed up by action, as the MHA sued the state; the administration capitulated and released the funds in an out-of-court settlement. In the end, however, health care providers received $488 million in overdue Medicaid payments and bad debt/free care allowances (Wallin 1994). After the Dukakis administration's attempt to "slow down" Medicaid reimbursement succumbed to the hospital industry's legal challenge, state officials turned to program reductions and sweeping cuts in other state programs in an effort to balance the budget.

Although the Weld administration proposed deep cuts in Medicaid funding as part of its fiscal austerity package in 1991, intergovernmental aid provided a "painless" solution to Massachusetts' budget woes. Using a narrow loophole first identified by an analyst in the state Medicaid program, Massachusetts collected $489 million in additional reimbursement from the U.S. Health Care Financing Administration to defray the cost of indigent care in what OMB Director Richard Darman denounced as a "scam" (Mashek and Phillips 1991). Disproportionate share hospital (DSH) payments accounted for 12.2% of total Medicaid expenditures in FY1993, netting the state more than $264 million in new intergovernmental revenues (Ku and Coughlin 1994). In an ironic turn of events, Medicaid offered a painless solution to Massachusetts' budgetary woes, for the state retained more than 45% of all new funds generated by provider taxes and federal matching payments (Kaiser Commission 1995). The federal aid windfall made the administration's threatened cutbacks in optional services unnecessary, but senior state officials soon indicated that a new strategy to control Medicaid costs was needed.

From the administration's point of view, uncontrollable spending on Medicaid was a function of an archaic and complex regulatory apparatus. Governor Weld vigorously endorsed a competitive solution to the state's health care cost crisis and sought to redefine the state's health policy agenda as the legislature began to consider its options for renewing the prospective rate-setting system created during the 1980s. In the eyes of the new Republican administration, unbridled competition among hospitals for a shrinking pool of patients coupled with aggressive use of managed care by Medicaid offered the best hope for controlling health care costs.

The commonwealth's efforts to grapple with its fiscal crises over the past two decades did not seriously challenge the fiscal health or decision-making autonomy of the hospital industry. In the 1970s, the hospital agreements approved by the Massachusetts Rate-Setting Commission were retrospective in nature, and fully reimbursed institutions for the cost of working capital, depreciation, bad debt, and charity care. The all-payer rate-setting system guaranteed hospitals an increase in revenue and created an uncompensated care pool to defray institutions' costs for free care and bad debts; since rates were based on institutions' historical costs, the system also implicitly rewarded inefficient institutions at the expense of efficient ones during the 1980s. Furthermore, although the state delayed payment of promised rate increases under HA-30 and HA-31, in the end state officials paid providers a negotiated settlement to avert a protracted court battle with the hospital industry. In short, state officials pursued a strategy of accommodation, rather than direct confrontation, in an effort to control rising health care costs.

The genesis of the all-payer rate-setting system in the early 1980s also reflects a consensus-building approach to health care policy-making. Chapter 372 emerged from a meso-corporatist bargaining process in which both policy formation and decision-making was delegated to a loose coalition of health insurers, providers, and state representatives assembled and held together by the power of business groups (Bergthold 1990b). Under a meso-corporatist system, bargaining takes place between state officials and powerful peak associations who wield the authority to act on behalf of their member institutions (Cawson 1986; Offe 1981). In addition, the state relied heavily on private groups to implement policy prior to the 1980s; more than half of the employees who worked for the MRSC were actually "on loan" from Blue Cross.

In 1982, the authorization for the all-payer system "was brokered not by the legislature itself but by an association of large private corporations, the Massachusetts Business Roundtable. Through the leadership of this organization, selected stakeholders were brought to the negotiating table and a solution was hammered out in private" (Bergthold 1988, 426). As one MRSC commissioner noted in 1990, "For a number of years the interested parties got together and said 'Let's try to reach some agreement on how hospitals should be paid.' They arrived at the legislature and said 'Here, adopt this because everyone who cares about it has already made the tradeoffs and is in agreement.'" Growing fissures in the coalition that had created the all-payer system, however, ensured that the state's quasi-corporatist approach to policy-making would be short-lived.

The influence of societal groups in health care decision-making during the early 1980s was enhanced by the commitment of the MBRT's chairman, Nelson Gifford, to health care reform. Gifford was able to arouse the interest of the state's business community in health care financing, activating a politically potent lobby on an issue that affected every business in the state. Gifford stepped into the leadership void in 1981 and 1982, bringing the disparate interests of Blue Cross, the hospitals, commercial insurers, and state officials together at the MBRT's offices in Waltham. When parties broke off negotiations, Gifford cajoled them to return to the table. Indeed, Bergthold (1990, 17) contends that Chapter 372 "occurred because Gifford made it a business decision-making process, not a public policy process." If the movement of health care debates "out of Boston and back to the offices of the MBRT in suburban Waltham, outside the beltway that rims Boston" (Bergthold 1988) had symbolic significance in 1982, the shift of venue to the legislature in 1987 and 1988 was equally significant.

After 1985, both legislators and affected interests expressed dissatisfaction with the closed bargaining process that gave birth to the all-payer system. In response to these criticisms, decisions affecting hospital reimbursement "went public" in the years that followed; in place of closed meetings between providers, insurers, and selected state officials, debates over health care financing featured extensive public hearings and press coverage, as well as pitched legislative battles between health insurers and the hospital industry. The increased visibility of legislative debates over health care, however, opened up the policy process to participation by new groups (Kronick 1990). By 1988, virtually everyone involved in health care financing had joined the debate, including advocates for the poor, public interest groups, labor, and proponents of universal health insurance. Representative Richard Voke, the chair of the House Ways and Means Committee, insisted that he had "never seen as many constituencies involved in a bill— never" (Knox 1987d, 86). As one commissioner described it,

> The arena has shifted to the Legislature . . . because with the escalating health care costs, everyone else is up there [on Beacon Hill]: business folks, small business folks, people trying to get a reduction in premiums. Everyone is up there and they're very strong and effective lobbying groups—they've hired former legislators to direct their activities.

The entry of new participants into policy debates over health care financing was accompanied by a new policy image for health care reform. Before 1987, health care policy-making in Massachusetts was defined by a concern over rising costs; after 1987, increasing access to care had displaced cost control as the primary concern for policymakers. This redefinition of policy goals had lasting consequences for the coalition which crafted the state's all-payer system. Businesses had entered the political arena in an effort to preserve competition in the state's health insurance market and control employee health care costs, not to expand social benefits.

Expanding health insurance to the uninsured had a powerful political appeal for legislators and the Dukakis administration. Although Governor Dukakis had initially proposed an incremental strategy to expand coverage through several regional pilot programs, the governor soon found himself on the defensive as legislators seized the limelight with proposals for comprehensive health care reform. The MHA had initially opposed universal health insurance, but hospitals successfully lobbied to delete provisions from the legislature's proposed hospital financing package that would have restricted hospital charges to 1% above the medical care component of the consumer price index. Hospitals' support for universal health insurance had a price: higher rates of reimbursement for all procedures, as well as favorable decisions to help hospitals with growing problems of uncompensated care and declining revenues for Medicare patients. Although the MHA failed in its bid to pass the bill in 1987, the end result was well worth the wait, for the pie got sweeter for the industry as time passed.

The Massachusetts Hospital Association pursued universal health care as a solution to hospitals' burgeoning financial exposure from uncompensated care. Without the industry's assent, attempts to pass either Senator Patricia McGovern's Massachusetts Health Partnership plan or the Dukakis administration's own reform proposals stalled in the Massachusetts legislature in 1987. The ensuing debate over universal health care underscored the enormous influence of the hospital industry, for most of the money that was pumped into the health care system in the late 1980s after the passage of Chapter 23 was not used for expanded access to health care, but rather for higher payments for existing services. Under the terms of HA-31, the new master contract for Blue Cross approved by the legislature, the state funnelled money to hospitals in the form of expanded bad debt and free care pools and a new Medicare shortfall assistance fund. Although these were never fully funded because of the state's fiscal crisis in 1989, they illustrate the political constraints facing public officials in Massachusetts. Hospital support for the plan was purchased through a massive infusion of public dollars to fund higher labor costs and rising expenses for bad debts and charity care. As one senior official at the MRSC recalled in 1990, "a lot of people feel that universal health care was bought with the changes in the hospital payment system. Because the other objective (universal health insurance) was to get a fairly controversial and fairly radical proposal in place, it gave the hospital association a lot of leverage to block it unless they got enough of what their membership was looking for."

DEREGULATION IN MASSACHUSETTS: REGIME CHANGE OR MORE OF THE SAME?

The coalition that supported Chapter 23 was more fragile than its creators realized. The state's ability to meet its obligations under the new system was suspect from the start, for the Dukakis administration had committed the state to an ambitious social program it could ill afford in a weak economy. Hospital support for the plan had been purchased through a massive infusion of public dollars to fund higher labor costs and rising expenses for bad debts and charity care. The state began to back out of its initial commitments as the true extent of its budget crisis became known, and the common interests uniting business, hospitals, and insurers quickly dissolved. Hospitals' efforts to secure the funds promised by the act proved unsuccessful. Less than a year after its passage, House members rejected $127 million in additional payments to the industry by a two-to-one margin and slashed funding for implementation of the new law to one-fifth of the level sought by the Dukakis administration (Mohl 1989a). By 1989, support for the universal health care law was wearing thin among legislators concerned about the state's rapidly deteriorating fiscal health. Richard Voke, the chair of the House Ways and Means Committee and a key supporter of the 1988 legislation, noted that "there's a lot of people who would repeal it if they had the opportunity" (quoted in Mohl 1989a, 38).

The fervor to deregulate the hospital industry took the Bay State by storm in less than a year's time. A year before the Weld administration's plan was endorsed by the legislature, MHA president Steven Hegarty argued that the industry "need[s] external discipline. We will work toward acceptable measures of external standards of efficiency. That can only be done in a . . . regulatory base" (quoted in Knox 1990a). These sentiments were echoed by the chair of the Massachusetts Rate Setting Commission, who felt that "businesses, the state, and the Hospital Association had surprisingly similar premises. . . . No one around the table is saying, as far as the immediate next step is concerned, that if we just get rid of government everything will be fine" (quoted in Knox 1990a, 24). In a burst of optimism, consumer groups such as Health Care For All enthused that "it's very heartening that people from such disparate positions are moving in the same direction. The left-wing and right-wing sectors are thinking in the same way: There has to be more public sector involvement. It can't be left to the private sector" (quoted in Knox 1990a, 24). The consensus over the need for continued state regulation, however, proved to be illusory; by the end of 1991, legislators, hospitals, and payers joined together in an unlikely coalition to end state regulatory controls over the hospital industry.

On the surface, the principal stakeholders in the state's health policy regime, with the exception of Blue Cross, supported the continuation of rate regulation in some form in 1990. Business groups have traditionally supported deregulation as a matter of principle, but the Associated Industries of Massachusetts (AIM) attacked the Weld deregulation plan on the grounds that it "appears to add to the inflationary spike which has punctuated health care costs in Massachusetts" (quoted in Knox 1991b). In place of deregulation, AIM called on its members to support a cap on acute-care hospital revenues as "the first essential requirement of any realistic hospital finance law." The *Boston Globe* also condemned the measure as "a risky gamble" that "is fraught with danger, including the potential for higher, rather than lower, hospital-payment rates" and urged legislators to extend the provisions of Chapter 23 until a suitable replacement could be found.

The push toward deregulation was made possible by the decision of top Democratic legislators to embrace competition as the cure for the commonwealth's health care ills. Support for the Weld administration's plan rose steadily throughout 1991; as the legislative session drew to a close, proponents included both co-chairs of the legislature's health care committee, the chair of the House Ways and Means Committee, and the co-chair of the House Insurance Committee (Knox 1991d). Few liberals remained committed to the ambitious program to control costs and increase access to health care through state regulation approved in 1988. One of the few dissenters, Representative John McDonough, complained that "you expect Republicans to push hard on deregulation, but you don't expect Democrats to capitulate to the Republican agenda without justification" (quoted in Hanafin 1991c). In a stunning turn-about from the previous year's consensus among providers, businesses, and consumer groups, the House approved the Weld administration's plan to deregulate hospital payment with few amendments by a 119–27 vote in late November (Hanafin 1991a); a last-minute proposal to substitute a single-payer plan introduced by John McDonough was soundly defeated. Boston's commissioner of health and hospitals, Judith Kurland, warned that under deregulation, "the whole health care system is going to fall apart. I think people know that and are going to let it happen" (quoted in Knox 1991c, 26).

Hospitals initially opposed deregulation on the grounds that it would exacerbate the industry's fiscal plight. In 1990, the MHA warned legislators of a continuing "fiscal crisis that confronts the hospital delivery system in Massachusetts" that had been fueled by the state's failure to fully fund the provisions of Chapter 23. In addition to ending the guarantee of hospital revenues through maximum allowable charges, Governor Weld's proposal to deregulate the payment system also marked the end of state funding for bad debts. Despite these losses, MHA president Steven Hegarty endorsed the law as "a balanced bill" that encouraged hospitals to deliver "the highest quality care at the lowest possible cost" (quoted in Britton 1992, NW6). As the MHA's spokesman explained, the amended bill "appears to be a thoughtful balance between competition and regulation" which involved "less micromananging. Most institutions will have the flexibility to stay within the cap" (quoted in Canellos 1991). Within the industry, support for the measure varied according to institutions' market position—while some hospitals in competitive markets offered discounts of up to 50% in order to win Blue Cross contracts, institutions with fewer competitors saw less to fear from the new law (Stein 1992). In particular, institutions that expected to gain patient volume applauded deregulation as a means of "evening the playing field" (Britton 1992).

Hospitals' change of heart reflected amendments to the bill in the House Ways and Means Committee that guaranteed full state reimbursement for free care and imposed a cap on hospital revenues. By ending restrictions on hospital rates, the plan also raised the de facto limits on hospital revenues established by the MRSC (Britton 1992); in the past, hospitals which had overbilled above their approved revenue ceiling had been forced to reimburse third-party insurers and/or patients for the full cost of their excess billing. Ignoring warnings that deregulation would boost hospital profits, legislators passed a modified version of the administration's proposal on the last day of the 1991 session.

The passage of Chapter 495 in 1991 revealed a striking ideological transformation within Massachusetts' health policy regime. The co-chairman of the legislature's Health Care Committee, Senator Edward Burke, was one of the principal supporters of Chapter 23 in 1988. In 1991, however, he was criticized by his fellow Democrats for "capitulating" to the Weld administration's demands to deregulate the hospital industry. The new policy-making climate in Massachusetts was evident in Burke's rebuttal to his critics:

> I planted the seed . . . for a lot of what the governor filed. . . . Just because we're Democrats doesn't mean that we stand for the continued presence of a large and complicated bureaucracy. I think our present apparatus for hospital regulation has been ineffective. The proof is in the pudding (quoted in Howe 1991).

The debate over deregulation also exposed the inherent contradictions in the state's health care policy-issue network. As the vice president of the Massachusetts Taxpayers Foundation observed in 1993, "The fiscal crisis has made it easier to make hard choices" (quoted in Stein 1993). Hospitals were initially reluctant to endorse deregulation because of the uncertainties associated with intense market competition. As the industry realized that most institutions would be able to increase their revenues in a deregulated system, however, hospitals warmed up to the administration's proposal. Blue Cross strongly supported the deregulation plan in the belief that selective contracting would save the company money and improve its ability to attract and retain subscribers.

Business groups faced a quandary with the Weld administration's proposals. Corporate leaders strongly supported the principle of market competition as a means to control costs, but were leery of hospitals using deregulation as a pretext to increase prices. After nearly a decade of comprehensive rate regulation, Massachusetts still led the nation in terms of per capita hospital expenditures. Hospital price increases, in turn, would raise the cost of employee fringe benefits. In the absence of a clear consensus on options for reform, the definition of the state's health policy agenda was left to the governor, who argued that "simplifying the regulatory process and enhancing competition could be vital to the future of the system. Certainly most would agree that the current system doesn't work very well" (quoted in Knox 1991a).

THE LIMITS OF STATE AUTONOMY IN MASSACHUSETTS

State officials in Massachusetts have operated under a broad legislative mandate to regulate the cost of health care services for more than two decades. In addition, during the 1980s, legislators authorized the expansion of state efforts to improve access to care for the poor and uninsured. The Massachusetts Rate-Setting Commission (MRSC) is authorized to review the reasonableness of all hospital payment rates in the commonwealth. The scope of the MRSC's authority is evident in the enabling legislation that created the all-payer system in 1982. Chapter 372 invested the commission with the power to "approve any rate of payment to any provider or class of providers if such rate, in the opinion of the commission, contains an incentive to achieve greater efficiency and economy in the manner of providing health care services without adversely affecting the quality of such services." These powers were expanded in subsequent years, as legislators authorized the creation of an Uncompensated Care Pool funded by an assessment on hospital charges, targeted funds to hospitals with "low base costs" and to institutions which were unduly affected by Medicare's adoption of a prospective payment system, and imposed new mandates on businesses and hospitals to provide health insurance and free care.

The broad scope of state power to regulate the hospital industry was routinely supported by the courts over the past two decades. Legal challenges to rate-setting methodology and capital expenditure controls in Massachusetts revolved around narrow issues of program implementation. Neither providers nor payers seriously challenged the legitimacy of state efforts to regulate hospital rates, fund uncompensated care, or review capital projects as a means to contain health care costs. The Supreme Judicial Court of Massachusetts upheld challenges to the MRSC's decision-making authority in a series of cases in the late 1980s and early 1990s. As the court noted in *Children's Hospital v. Rate Setting Commission* in 1991, HA-30 granted the MRSC "significant discretionary authority" to determine adjustments or exceptions to the computation of maximum allowable costs for individual hospitals. The MRSC had denied Children's Hospital's appeal for additional reimbursement to cover higher labor costs in 1987, despite the hospital's claim that its shortage of nurses constituted an "unusual and extraordinary occurrence" that qualified for an exemption under the terms of HA-30. In rejecting the hospital's appeal, the court argued that the MRSC's position was "both reasonable and in accord with the policy of cost containment" embodied in the enabling legislation. In two related cases in 1990, the court upheld the MRSC's denial of Emerson Hospital's request for additional operating funds associated with an ongoing renovation and expansion project and rejected a challenge to the commission's settlement procedures for disbursing uncompensated care funds.[8]

Despite this mandate to pursue a regulatory strategy to control health care costs, state officials have been unable to impose restrictive cost-containment policies on recalcitrant providers and payers over the past two decades. In part, the accommodative nature of the commonwealth's cost-containment initiatives reflect the economic impact and political effectiveness of industry groups; legislators have been wary of undermining the fiscal health of a vital and growing component of the Massachusetts economy. In addition, policymakers' efforts to foster competition among providers were also hampered by institutional constraints. With few exceptions, persistent infighting over health care financing between the executive branch and the legislature diminished the coherence and consistency of state cost-control policies. Frequent clashes over authority, goals, and strategies among public agencies in Massachusetts made it difficult to conceive of the state as a unitary actor pursuing a consistent policy agenda. The resulting discord among public officials provided numerous opportunities to pit government actors against each other in struggles over turf and blunted the effectiveness of the state's efforts to control health care costs.

The Legislature

The Massachusetts legislature has been staunchly Democratic in recent decades; Republicans were outnumbered by a margin of four to one throughout the 1980s in both chambers. Indeed, Democrats have controlled both houses of the Massachusetts legislature since 1959. Republicans nearly doubled their strength in the Senate in the 1990 election by winning 15 of the 40 seats and providing the state's newly elected governor, William Weld, with enough support to sustain a veto. Republican success in legislative elections, however, proved to be short-lived, as Democrats reclaimed veto-proof majorities in both chambers in 1992. Democrats solidified their control in both 1994 and 1996; at the start of the 1997 legislative session, Republicans were outnumbered by a 34–6 margin in the Senate and 131–29 in the House. In the face of continued Democratic dominance of the legislature, the Weld administration has been forced to compromise with the Democratic leadership in order to achieve its goal of reducing the size and scope of the state government. Power in the legislature is also highly centralized. In addition to assigning members to committees and selecting committee chairs, nearly all decisions in the House and Senate, from office space and staff to parking, are controlled by their presiding officers (Berg 1993).

Lawmakers in Massachusetts work in one of the most professional state legislatures in the nation. All members are assigned office space and year-round personal staff. In addition, while legislative service remains a part-time job for most members, service pays well relative to other state legislatures; the annual salaries of lawmakers in Massachusetts rose from $12,688 in 1977 to $30,000 in 1994. Members also benefit from both clerical and professional staff assigned to the legislature's standing committees. Legislative turnover in recent years has been below the national average; after the November 1994 elections, only 15% of the Senate was comprised of new legislators, while in the House 16.3% of members were freshmen representatives. Further evidence of growing professionalization appeared in a 1992 study by the National Conference of State Legislatures, which categorized Massachusetts as one of only nine state legislatures in the U.S. to exhibit the characteristics of a full-time legislature in terms of salaries, staffing, and the length of the legislative session (Jones 1995).

The interest groups that descended upon the legislature to lobby for universal health insurance in 1987 and 1988 were greeted by a cadre of policy entrepreneurs and legislative leaders who were deeply interested in health care reform. The growing sophistication and interest of legislators in health care financing was particularly evident during the debate over universal health insurance in 1988, when members debated the intricacies of the master contract between Blue Cross and participating hospitals over a period of several months. Legislative debate during 1987 and 1988 explored the impact of volume incentives, labor add-ons, and a wide range of minutiae that had previously been the province of the MRSC or left to the discretion of Blue Cross officials. The extensive debate over Chapter 23 in 1988 served notice that Massachusetts legislators were willing to assert themselves on health care policy-making matters rather than merely taking cues from the health bureaucracy and key interest groups. As the chair of the MRSC explained in 1990,

> Chapter 372 got passed with very little debate in the House and the Senate. All the parties agreed, so the legislature didn't think much about it. In this last go-around with Chapter 23 you had legislators offering totally new amendments and new bills.

These developments reflect the increasing professionalism in state legislatures generally over the past two decades; members now take their roles as policy entrepreneurs seriously, not unlike their counterparts in Congress (see Loomis 1988). As Senator Edward Burke, the long-time co-chair of the legislature's joint Health Care Committee, related in 1991, "what keeps me going is this health care stuff. I'm a junkie. I love this stuff. There's no more interesting thing that the legislature deals with. I still have a zest for the fray" (quoted in Knox 1991c, 26). Senator Patricia McGovern's role as an issue entrepreneur in health care financing debates in 1987 and 1988 also illustrates the steady growth of legislative interest and involvement in health care financing. McGovern was the strongest and best-known legislative supporter of universal health care; the introduction of her comprehensive universal health insurance proposal (the Massachusetts Health Partnership) redefined the agenda for health care reform several months before the Dukakis administration fully endorsed the concept.[9] As one former director of the MRSC's Bureau of Hospitals observed in 1990,

> Over the past ten years the legislature has become more involved and more influential in [determining] what the final product is going to look like. It used to be that the legislature would set a final policy and the Commission would say "here's how we're going to do that." Now you've got the legislature saying "here's how you're going to do it" and leaving less flexibility for the interpretation of the law.

Despite the flurry of interest in health care financing during the 1980s, Democratic legislators failed to challenge the Weld administration's proposal to deregulate the hospital industry in 1991. While some observers attributed the passivity of legislators to a growing sense of burnout after years of grappling with intractable policy issues, the *Boston Globe* editorialized that "the Legislature is likely to approve the new method because few legislators understand any part of it and because the Massachusetts Hospital Association is going along with it" (*Boston Globe* 1991). In a remarkable about-face, even some of the legislature's most experienced and active policy entrepreneurs on health care issues embraced the Weld plan. Senator Edward Burke told colleagues that he favored "putting the scorpions in the same bottle . . . and letting them fight it out" (quoted in Knox 1991c, 26).

Legislative politics may change in the coming years as a result of the passage of term limits in 1994. In other states that have adopted term limits, departures from the legislature increased substantially even before members were required to leave their positions (Rosenthal 1996). Recent scandals and turnover in the senior leadership of the Massachusetts House and Senate have also contributed to an unsettled policy-making environment. In 1996, Senate President William Bulger resigned to become president of the University of Massachusetts, while his counterpart in the House, Speaker Charles Flaherty, was forced to leave office in disgrace.

The Governor

Each of Massachusetts' governors over the past two decades became actively involved in health care regulation and reform, but their incentives for involvement differed. In the early 1980s, Governor Ed King was dragged into the debate over hospital financing at the behest of business groups and industry officials. As Linda Bergthold (1988, 430) argued, "Governor King chose to defuse the conflict [over hospital rate increases] by persuading the MRSC chairman and staff to put a freeze on hospital charges and to cap the rates of increase until a new study commission . . . could come up with recommendations acceptable to all parties." If King was an interest broker mediating disputes among warring factions, Governor Michael Dukakis played the role of a policy entrepreneur who eagerly pushed health care reform. Although Dukakis deferred to the business community that had forged agreement over Chapter 372 again in 1985 when Chapter 574 was renegotiated, the governor and his staff appropriated the cause of universal access early in 1988. With the impending disaster facing the state's economy still more than a year off, Dukakis embraced the cause of universal health care with vigor.

William Weld became the first Republican to win the governorship in twenty years when he edged John Silber, the controversial president of Boston University, with 50.2% of the vote in 1990. Weld was easily re-elected in 1994. Although Weld entered office with an ambitious agenda to reinvent and downsize state government, his proposals were frequently stonewalled by the Democratically controlled legislature. Upon entering office, Weld faced an extraordinary fiscal crisis—the state faced a deficit of more than $850 million in FY1991 despite tax increases in FY1989 and FY1990. Wall Street investment firms had downgraded the state's bond rating twice, and unless the state put its fiscal house in order, the state's credit rating was expected to fall to "junk bond" status (Hale 1992; Wallin 1995). Since Weld adamantly refused to increase taxes in order to balance the budget, massive budget cuts were inevitable; more than 300 programs suffered cuts during the FY1991 and FY1992 budget negotiations, netting a savings of more than $800 million in FY1991 and $1.8 billion in FY1992 (Wallin 1995).

During the 1990 campaign and in his first months in office, Weld vigorously pushed his vision of "entrepreneurial government" as a means of providing public services to Massachusetts residents more efficiently and at a lower cost. On the campaign trail in 1990, Weld promised to "move in the direction of a more competitive [health care] industry" and pledged to "take the regulatory wraps off health care" if elected (quoted in Knox 1990a, 24). For the Weld administration, the deregulation of hospital prices represented one battle in a much larger war for the soul of state government in Massachusetts. In a widely discussed plan for downsizing Massachusetts state government introduced in 1995, Weld argued that "the solution is not simply to spend less. Government ought not do more with less—it ought to do less with less" (Weld and Cellucci 1995, 7). The pledge was not idle rhetoric, for despite the legislature's resistance to the governor's plans to reorganize state government, Weld pressed ahead with plans to reduce the state code of regulations by roughly 20%. The Rate Setting Commission emerged as one of the principal targets of the governor's effort to cut red tape. The regulatory reform effort spearheaded by Finance Secretary Charles Baker, Jr., proposed to eliminate 34 of the 89 regulations issued by the MRSC and modify 48 others; only 7 regulations would be retained in their present form (Grunwald 1996).

After winning reelection to a second term by a comfortable majority in 1994, Weld reiterated his call for changing the role of government. Government, according to Weld, "should not meddle in the market. Government should not 'pick' winners by substituting the judgment of state planners for the market of private individuals" (Weld and Cellucci 1995, 12). In particular, the governor and his aides vigorously opposed the employer mandate which was the cornerstone of Dukakis' universal health insurance program. Under the provisions of the 1988 legislation, all employers were required to either provide a basic health insurance package for their workers or contribute to a state-managed health insurance pool. Philip Johnston, Dukakis' secretary of human services, argued that legislative repeal of this provision "would essentially gut the law." Weld did not disagree with this assessment, and urged the legislature to repeal both the employer mandate and the state's prospective rate-setting system. The administration also sought to fundamentally redefine the way Massachusetts provides medical care to the poor by imposing a "managed care" framework upon the state's Medicaid program. By 1996, more than 400,000 program beneficiaries had signed up with a health maintenance organization or selected a primary care provider from an approved network of physicians and community health centers.

The Bureaucracy

Although the Massachusetts Rate-Setting Commission (MRSC) was at the center of health care regulation during the 1970s and 1980s, its policy-making role has receded over time. Few formal mechanisms exist to coordinate the activities of state regulatory agencies in Massachusetts. Each of the departments and commissions involved in health care financing—the Executive Office of Human Services, the state Medicaid program, and the Department of Public Health's Determination of Need (DON) program—has "almost complete operational autonomy" (Kinney 1987, 410). In addition, turnover in key policy-making positions has been high in state regulatory agencies, as many senior executives and analysts sought higher pay and better working conditions in the private sector.

The changes in the MRSC preceded, and in many ways precipitated, major changes in the state's hospital reimbursement policies. The MRSC was created in 1968, when the legislature consolidated two smaller agencies—the Bureau of Hospital Costs and a rate-setting commission for nursing homes—into a single agency. The commission's authorizing legislation empowered it to establish "fair, reasonable and adequate rates" for all health care providers operating in the commonwealth. The commission was relatively insulated from the state's budgetary woes in the 1970s because its operating expenses were funded by an assessment on hospitals. The commission was also shaped by its close relationship with Blue Cross and Blue Shield of Massachusetts; before 1982 more than 80 of its auditors were employed by Blue Cross and "lent" to the MRSC. The reason for this peculiar arrangement was simple—both the MRSC and Blue Cross were required to audit hospitals to determine appropriate reimbursement rates for providers. Since Blue Cross needed to conduct its own audits, assigning some of its personnel to the MRSC enabled the commission to avoid unnecessary duplication of staff. The passage of the all-payer system in 1982, however, ended this arrangement.

Prior to 1982, the commission operated with considerable autonomy as a *rate-setting* body with substantial rule-making powers. As one commissioner noted in 1990, under Chapter 409 the MRSC had the "authority to develop regulations under which hospitals were to be regulated; there was a lot more discretion given to the agency at that time." Although the MRSC supported the concept of an all-payer system in 1981, its genesis with the passage of Chapter 372 in 1982 moved the commission from center stage in hospital reimbursement policy-making to a more peripheral role. The commission was conspicuous by its absence during the bargaining process that produced Chapter 372. As the chair of the MRSC noted in 1990, "Ever since Chapter 372 the administrative discretion of the state in regulating hospital rates has been severely limited. It's much more defined by statute now; the commission has been much more the administrator of the system rather than its designer."

In effect, Chapter 372 and its successors spelled out the terms of the Blue Cross master contract in statute, leaving the commission with few formal responsibilities for determining the rate of reimbursement for hospitals. Although dissatisfied institutions have occasionally challenged the MRSC's decisions in court, few of the commission's rulings have been overturned on appeal.

High staff turnover at the MRSC in the late 1980s and early 1990s made even daily administrative responsibilities, let alone policy development, an onerous task. As one Blue Cross vice president observed in 1990, "The fallout from the political instability at the rate-setting commission has been turnover. A lot of people who'd been there for a number of years left and now you're left with people who haven't been there trying to learn the system." Numerous exceptions and modifications to the MAC methodology, however, made it difficult for a newcomer to learn in a short span of time. Constant turnover within the MRSC's Hospital Bureau ensured that some personnel were always "learning the ropes." As one former director of the Bureau of Hospitals recalled,

> Turnover in general is fairly high—20–30% per year . . . Once you get good at the Commission, you can pretty much name your own terms. Although the benefits package with the state is fantastic, the pay is not

competitive. A person who worked for the Commission as an analyst for three years could expect to make $15–20,000 more a year in the private sector. People leave because the Commission is a wonderful place to learn new skills and then get employed by industry . . . the [hospital] industry pays much better.

The dire fiscal straits Massachusetts faced in the late 1980s and early 1990s provided a strong incentive for many of the state's most talented administrators to leave; by 1990, raises for the MRSC's staff were more than two years overdue. In addition, statewide hiring freezes in 1989 and 1990 made it impossible to replace staff members who left the commission. Paul Swaboda, the Hospital Bureau's director in the early 1980s, left to form his own consulting business. Another bureau director, Steven Tringale, left the commission for a position with the Life Insurance Association of Massachusetts; he currently works as a senior executive for Blue Cross and Blue Shield of Massachusetts. The bureau's director in the mid-1980s, John Chapman, left in 1988 for a position in the newly created Department of Medical Security, which was given the challenge of implementing the Dukakis administration's universal health insurance scheme. Chapman's successor, Richard Michel, left the MRSC to work on health care financing issues for the accounting firm of Coopers and Lybrand. The consequences of such a high turnover rate among key personnel were clear and immediate. As one commissioner noted in 1990,

We've lost several key managers, and we've lost a bit of that institutional grooming. It's related to a lot of things, including state worker bashing. These are talented folks, and we've never had anyone leave here who went to a job that paid less money. We asked Rich [Michel] if we could keep him; he asked if we could double his salary. The marketplace is so competitive that when you get someone with his skills, they're in demand.

Similar fiscal crises faced other state agencies in the late 1980s and early 1990s. The state's FY1990 budget failed to provide sufficient funding to hire the twenty staff positions authorized for the newly created Department of Medical Security charged with implementing Massachusetts' universal health insurance program (Knox 1989a).

TENSIONS WITHIN MASSACHUSETTS' HEALTH POLICY REGIME

Health care policy-making in Massachusetts continues to be defined by constant sparring among the principal players in the state's negotiated policy regime. Cost control remains an important issue in the Bay State, but as a result of growing competition among hospitals for patients and the successful implementation of the state's Medicaid managed care waiver, concerns over costs no longer dominate the health policy agenda. Indeed, sharp declines in the AFDC caseload, coupled with the state's ability to bargain for volume discounts with providers, have brought Medicaid expenditures down to manageable levels despite recent expansions of eligibility under the terms of the state's Section 1115 waiver. Since business groups have also been able to manage their costs without state assistance by forming purchasing alliances and shifting costs to their employees, the sense of urgency which accompanied health care policy-making in the 1980s was notably absent by the 1990s.

The principal tensions in Massachusetts' health care policy regime reflect the changing nature of health care organization and financing in the commonwealth. Policymakers remain committed to improving access without resorting to an employer mandate. In addition, concerns over the financing of uncompensated care remain a contentious issue between hospitals and third-party payers; legislative leaders have promised to explore options for revamping the state's uncompensated care pool during 1997. Finally, the rapid pace of consolidation within the Massachusetts hospital industry in recent years brought new calls for expanded state oversight of hospital mergers, particularly in cases where for-profit hospital chains seek to acquire nonprofit institutions.

Despite the rollback of state regulation of the hospital industry in the early 1990s, Massachusetts remains committed to expanding access to health care for the uninsured. The employer mandate, a cornerstone of the state's plan to provide universal health insurance for Massachusetts residents, was scheduled to take effect in 1991. Legislators postponed the implementation deadline twice before repealing it in 1996. Although the legislative leadership had endorsed the plan in 1988, by 1994 leading Democrats such as Representative Carmen Buell, the co-chair of the legislature's joint health care committee, argued that the mandate could place the state at a "serious economic disadvantage by placing added costs on business" (quoted in Wong 1994, 37). In 1994, Attorney General Scott Harshbarger entered the fray, calling for new public standards on "community benefits" provided by nonprofit hospitals; institutions that failed to meet the state guidelines would risk losing their tax-exempt status. Under the proposal, hospitals would be required to provide community benefits equal to the value of their tax exemption or up to 7% of their patient care expenses (Knox 1994a). MHA president Steven Hegarty assailed the proposal as an effort to "revert back to a regulatory approach which is out of step with the direction we believe the health care system is headed" (quoted in Knox 1994a).

With the approval of the Weld administration's Medicaid managed care waiver application in 1995, new state initiatives to increase access to care for the uninsured were assured. Haggling over the exact nature of such initiatives, however, and the appropriate means of financing expanded access, produced a year-long standoff between the governor and the legislative leaders. In July 1996, legislators overrode a Weld veto of a plan that expanded Medicaid eligibility to include 124,000 previously uninsured residents, extended health insurance coverage to 150,000 uninsured children, and prescription drug coverage to 65,000 low-income elderly adults (McDonough, Hager, and Rosman 1997). Although the Weld administration had opposed the 25-cent tax on cigarettes used to finance the measure, the measure passed in the House by a margin of 115 to 42; the Senate easily overrode the governor's veto by a margin of 30 to 6. In a significant departure from past practice, the legislation (Chapter 203 of 1996) replaced categorical eligibility requirements for Medicaid with a simple income threshold that offered coverage to residents with household incomes of less than 133% of the federal poverty line who did not have employer-sponsored insurance (McDonough, Hager, and Rosman 1997).

In a related issue, the adequacy of the state's uncompensated care pool has been contested since the passage of Chapter 495 in 1991. The MHA sued the Dukakis administration in 1990 after state officials placed limits on the amount of bad debt that qualified for reimbursement from the state's uncompensated care pool, funded through a surcharge on hospital charges. State funding for uncompensated care has remained frozen at FY1992 levels for four years. Since 1991, state funding for the free care pool has been capped at $315 million; at the same time, the assessment on hospital charges which fund the pool has declined from 13% to 8%. As a result, the percentage of indigent care costs reimbursed by Massachusetts' free care pool fell from 94% in 1992 to less than 65% in 1995 (Canellos 1995). Blue Cross' new contract with participating hospitals included payments for uncompensated care in the negotiated payments to hospitals. As the company noted in a full page ad in the *Boston Globe* in 1996, "It is the Massachusetts acute care hospitals who are legally obligated to provide uncompensated care and to make payments to the pool. It is not, and never has been, our responsibility."

Funding for the pool remains unresolved, for while hospitals provided more than $520 million in free care in 1996, private sector contributions to the pool remained capped at $315 million, resulting in a net loss for the industry of more than $200 million (Stein 1996b). Hospitals also assailed subsequent proposals to tap the pool to finance expanded coverage under the state's Medicaid managed care waiver. The MHA denounced the Weld administration's plan to draw more than $200 million from the pool, arguing that the "hospital is facing a crisis and it needs to be strengthened, not weakened" (quoted in Murphy 1996). The MHA estimated that full funding of the pool would require approximately $480 million in 1996 and continued to seek a commitment from legislators to redesign the financing of the pool so that costs are evenly distributed among hospitals, insurers, and the state. Businesses, however, have strongly opposed proposals to increase the surcharge on private insurance bills to raise revenues for the pool.

The extraordinary upheaval within the Massachusetts health care system in recent years presents an additional set of challenges for health care policymakers, for hospitals' desire to increase their efficiency and competitiveness through vertical and horizontal integration has drawn fire from consumer groups, local governments, and legislative delegations in affected communities—and from the attorney general's office. In 1993, the Senate Committee on Post Audit and Oversight called for more extensive state reviews of hospital mergers and consolidations after a ten-month investigation (Knox 1993). The Massachusetts Hospital Association, however, cautioned against "placing new roadblocks in the way of efforts by hospitals and others to collaborate to deliver health care more efficiently" (quoted in Knox 1993). By 1996, the entry of for-profit hospital chains into the Massachusetts health care system prompted public health commissioner David Mulligan to issue new regulations requiring for-profit chains to maintain the existing level of free care after purchasing nonprofit hospitals (Kong and O'Neill 1996).

Legislators have also shown considerable interest in establishing a public review process to evaluate the impact of proposed mergers on access to care, particularly where service consolidations are concerned. Establishing a comprehensive review process for mergers, however, threatens the managerial autonomy of the hospital industry. Of particular concern to the MHA and its members are proposals to require institutions to disclose the valuation of nonprofit hospitals and their "charitable assets" as a condition of obtaining state approval for proposed mergers.

CONCLUSION

Health care policy-making in Massachusetts continues to be governed by a negotiated regime, for while the state has turned to the market as a means to control costs, the administrative structure and statutory authority of state agencies remains intact. As Krasner (1978) and Ikenberry (1988) have observed in other policy arenas, the pursuit of a market-oriented strategy by public officials often provides an effective route to achieving state objectives. Without support from private groups, however, the state was unable to implement stringent price controls in an increasingly competitive health care marketplace. Although Massachusetts created one of the most heavily regulated hospital payment systems in the nation in the 1980s, the state's rate-setting system was less effective in controlling costs than in controlling cost shifting among payers.

While policymakers succeeded in creating a strong legislative mandate in support of hospital cost-containment, pressure from interest groups, particularly the Massachusetts Hospital Association, prevented the state from implementing more restrictive payment policies in the 1980s. Passage of universal health insurance was made possible by promises of additional revenues for the state's hospital industry; when the state failed to meet its obligations, hospitals pressed for relief—first in the courts, where the MHA's efforts led to a compromise on past due Medicaid payments, and later in the legislature, where lawmakers passed a deregulation plan in 1991 with the blessing of the MHA and third-party payers. The common interest among public and private participants in controlling cost shifting and promoting competition among hospitals which led to the creation of the all-payer system had faded by the late 1980s. By 1990, the principal stakeholders in Massachusetts' health policy regime jockeyed for position in an increasingly competitive environment.

Massachusetts' experience with hospital reimbursement in the 1980s illustrates how vulnerable political institutions can be to changes in leadership. The political leadership that forged the Bay State's regulatory orientation was never adequately institutionalized; the consensus forged by Nelson Gifford in 1982 evaporated as key players and the locus of decision-making moved to the legislature. As both the hospital industry and health insurers battled for the support of the business community, businesses were torn between their desire to lower health care costs and the appeal of high-quality health services. The end result was a severe case of cognitive dissonance, in which businesses' most prudent course of action was to withdraw from the debate altogether. Health care policy-making in Massachusetts offers a clear example of the limits of state autonomy, for state officials were unable to implement effective cost-control policies over the objections of the hospital industry once the public-private partnership which created Chapter 372 had dissolved.

Continuing tensions within Massachusetts' health policy regime have not reduced support for state intervention to curb the excesses of the marketplace. A careful review of past state efforts to regulate the behavior of the hospital industry, however, casts doubt upon the ability of pubic officials to impose significant restrictions on providers. The state, in short, lacks the ability to enforce its preferences in the face of concentrated resistance from societal groups.

CHAPTER NOTES

1. See Andrepoulous (1997) for an incisive critique of the recent wave of mergers among teaching hospitals.

2. Ross and Bright (1996) provide a comprehensive discussion of the merger and its consequences.

3. In 1996, for example, Digital employees typically paid $20 per week for HMO coverage, $30 per week for a point-of-service plan, and $175 per week for standard indemnity coverage. The result, not surprisingly, was a mass migration of employees to managed care plans. Enrollment in indemnity plans fell from 78% in 1990 to 7% in 1995, while managed care enrollment increased from 27.3% to more than 80% in the same period.

4. Medicaid paid providers on a prospective per diem basis for inpatient services; rates were computed by dividing total "allowable patient costs" in the base year by total inpatient days in the base year, and the resulting "per diem" rate was trended two years to the "rate" year by applying an industry-wide inflation factor (Esposito et al. 1982, 145). Reimbursement for charge payers under Chapter 409 continued on a retrospective basis. Prior to 1982, Blue Cross reimbursed hospitals based on the lower of reasonable costs or charges.

5. As Kronick (1990, 892) notes, "The 409 system was not effective at controlling either hospital costs or charges; worse, from the commercial insurers' point of view, even if the system did work to contain costs, there would be no guarantee that charges to commercial insurers would be restrained. The charge based payers were responsible for paying for the difference between the [Massachusetts] Rate-Setting Commission's definition of reasonable financial requirements and the reimbursement received from other payers."

6. HA-29 determined hospitals' reimbursement, known as the basis of payment (BOP), using two distinct components: maximum allowable costs (MAC) and annualized cost pass-throughs. The basis of payment for individual hospitals was computed by inflating approved charges (maximum allowable costs) in 1981 by a prenegotiated percentage for each year of the contract, adjusting for changes in volume, and adding in pass-through costs for capital expenditures or large shifts in an institution's case mix. Unlike the MAC, however, capital costs, free care/bad debts, and other pass-throughs were not prospectively budgeted, but instead were dropped from the computations each year and added in for the next year based upon actual incurred costs.

7. Under HA-30, hospitals received 50% of the marginal cost for each additional CMAD. One senior Blue Cross official recalled that "the hospitals argu[ed] that they were always getting a marginal adjustment, but what they

really needed was to start off square again—to be even with other hospitals. They got the difference between the [50%] marginal rate and 100% [volume variability under HA-31] added into their base. Both that and the low base cost adjustment were large."

8. See the court's arguments in *Emerson Hospital v. Rate Setting Commission* 562 N.E.2d 681 (Mass. 1990) and *The General Hospital Corporation v. Rate Setting Commission* 552 N.E. 2d 113 (Massachusetts 1990) for additional evidence that the legitimacy of state regulatory powers was not in question at the time Massachusetts opted to deregulate hospital charges.

9. McGovern's plan preempted the report of Dukakis' special commission on health care, chaired by Secretary of Human Services Philip Johnston and co-sponsored by the MBRT, which suggested a more cautious approach that proposed funding two pilot universal health insurance experiments that would cover 25,000 people in Worcester County and an additional 10,000 in Suffolk County.

5

Rhode Island:
Conflict and Collaboration in a
Negotiated Regime

"In Rhode Island we have a tradition of nonprofit health care and community hospitals. Our regulation and control is minimal, and much gets done based on trust and years of working together. . . ."
Lt. Governor Robert Weygand, 1996.

Health care policy-making in Rhode Island is governed by a negotiated policy regime with a strong corporatist flavor. Cooperation, not conflict, is the most prominent characteristic of the system. Although tensions exist among the participants in the state's health care financing system, neither hospitals nor third-party payers have pressed for significant changes in Rhode Island's unique rate-setting methodology (known as the "Maxicap") since its inception in the early 1970s. Although the state's certificate-of-need process has undergone considerable change since the mid-1980s, the Maxicap continues to enjoy strong support from hospitals, state officials, and third-party payers. In addition, Rhode Island's successful application for a Section 1115 Medicaid waiver has not changed the fundamental nature of its cost-control strategy, which is based on negotiation among the major stakeholders in the state's health care policy-issue network.

Private or quasi-public solutions to rising health care costs are the norm in Rhode Island. No underlying consensus among participants in the state's health care policy-issue network exists to support significant expansions of public authority, particularly when they threaten the interests of health care providers. The hospital industry has steadfastly opposed efforts to increase the scope of state regulatory powers over hospital reimbursement and capital expenditures. The state's preference for "public-private partnerships" to address policy problems has contributed to the development of a weak regulatory apparatus. As a

136

result, state agencies lack both statutory authority and resources to modify the behavior of providers. In the end, public authority over the hospital industry in Rhode Island is sharply circumscribed by the limited capacity of state political institutions, the presence of a well-organized and well-funded industry, and by continuing ambivalence over the dual role of hospitals as both employers and a source of continued health care inflation.

Even though tensions exist within Rhode Island's health policy regime, providers, third-party payers, and the state remain satisfied with the design and performance of the state's cost-containment strategy. Despite modest changes in the rules and decision-making process in recent years, the relationship between state officials and private groups in health care policy-making has changed little over two decades. In addition, health care policy-making has not been a subject of partisan or ideological conflict in Rhode Island. Instead, disputes largely reflect dissatisfaction with the state's certificate-of-need process and occasional conflicts over the fiscal impact of state aid and provider taxes on individual hospitals. Legal challenges to specific CON decisions have not led to efforts to change the state's unique reimbursement process, but rather relate to the interpretation of existing statutory mandates.

THE POLICY-MAKING ENVIRONMENT IN RHODE ISLAND

A small state with a population of just over one million people in 1990, Rhode Island is home to eleven acute-care hospitals, four of which are located in the capital city of Providence. Rhode Island's hospitals are a major force in the state's economy, as one of every nine workers in the state is employed in the health care industry. In 1994, hospitals employed more than 23,000 people; Rhode Island Hospital was the state's largest private employer. By the end of 1995, the majority of the state's hospitals had aligned themselves with one of two competing health care networks. Led by Rhode Island Hospital, several teaching hospitals affiliated with Brown University's School of Medicine formed Lifespan, an integrated delivery system that includes six acute-care hospitals, the state's largest visiting nurse service, and a children's psychiatric hospital. In early 1997 Lifespan acquired New England Medical Center, one of Boston's leading teaching hospitals and affiliated with Newport Hospital to create the first interstate hospital network in New England (Krieger and Rau 1997). In response to this move, three other hospitals banded together in 1995 to form Care New England. Four community hospitals remained unaffiliated with either network; although the sale of Roger Williams Medical Center to

Columbia/HCA was announced by the hospital's board of trustees in 1996, final approval of the purchase by the Department of Health and the state attorney general's office remained unresolved more than six months after the parties announced their merger plans.

Over the past two decades the Hospital Association of Rhode Island (HARI) has emerged as one of the state's most influential lobbying groups; paid lobbyists develop and track legislation affecting its membership, testify at hearings, and coordinate grass-roots campaigns with the association's member hospitals. HARI's political advantages were strengthened by the fact that until 1994 the 150 members of Rhode Island's legislature served only part-time and received only five dollars a day for their efforts. With little professional staff support available to individual members or committees, legislators relied heavily on testimony provided by interested parties in formulating legislation (Hyde 1993). Furthermore, local legislative delegations supported hospitals in light of their dual role as "charitable institutions" providing free care to the medically indigent and as major employers in local communities.

Prior to the mid-1980s, Rhode Island's hospital industry had not witnessed the intense competition that accompanied the expansion of for-profit hospital chains, managed care, and alternative delivery systems elsewhere. Blue Cross and Blue Shield of Rhode Island dominated the state's private health insurance market, capturing the highest market share of any Blue Cross plan in the nation by the late 1970s (Goldberg and Greenberg 1995). Blue Cross was also a founding partner of the state's prospective rate-setting program that determined both individual hospital budgets and an overall ceiling on hospital expenditures each year. Further, no preferred provider organizations operated in the state during the 1980s, and none entered the market in the early 1990s. Nevertheless, the merger of Roger Williams Medical Center to Columbia/HCA and Landmark Medical Center's continued interest in affiliating with OrNda or another for-profit chain suggest that the era of stability in Rhode Island's health care system is drawing to a close.

Competition among health care providers and third-party insurers for market share has increased dramatically in Rhode Island over the past decade. Membership in alternative delivery systems rose exponentially from fewer than 19,000 in 1975 to more than 222,000 in 1990. By 1993, Rhode Island had the eighth highest HMO market penetration in the nation, with more than 27% of the population enrolled in managed care (Marion Merrill Dow 1994). The intensified competition for paying patients, however, was not accompanied by the introduction of new health care providers. While four ambulatory surgical centers were licensed in Rhode Island during the 1980s, two were limited to providing abortion services and gynecological surgery. Until the proposed acquisition of Roger Williams Medical Center by Columbia/ HCA in 1996, no for-profit hospitals or national hospital chains operated in Rhode Island.

As the state's dominant third-party health insurer, Blue Cross held more than 70% of the nongovernment health insurance market in Rhode Island in the early 1990s. This occurred despite inroads by the state's two largest health maintenance organizations, United Health Care (formerly Ocean State Physicians Health Plan) and Harvard Community Health Plan of New England (formerly the Rhode Island Group Health Association). Blue Cross' aggressive response to the entry of Ocean State Physicians Health Plan (OSPHP) in the 1980s led to charges that the company employed unfair competitive practices in order to preserve its monopoly over the state's health insurance market (Goldberg and Greenberg 1995). In particular, the refusal of Blue Cross to pay participating physicians more than the lowest rate they would accept from other insurers and its decision to offer a new health insurance product (HealthMate) modeled after OSPHP's benefit package produced a lengthy legal battle in state and federal courts. Although both the U.S. District Court and the U.S. Court of Appeals rejected claims that the company had violated the provisions of the Sherman Antitrust Act in *Ocean State Physicians Health Plan v. Blue Cross*, competing HMOs did not need the courts to shore up their position, for both Ocean State and RIGHA continued to gain members throughout the 1980s. Given Blue Cross' relatively late move into managed care and other selective contracting arrangements, the Maxicap offered the company a legally binding process which institutionalized its leverage over the state's acute-care hospitals in a changing health care marketplace.[1]

Most conspicuous by its absence in health care policy-making is the business community. The principal advocate for the businesses' health care agenda has been the Rhode Island Business Group on Health (RIBGH), an organization founded by twenty of the state's largest companies. Despite these resources, however, the RIBGH, with one full-time staff member who doubles as both the organization's executive director and principal lobbyist, has not played a role in the state's rate-setting or certificate-of-need processes. Since the prospective payment system is linked to annual contract negotiations between Blue Cross and the state's hospitals, the decision-making and implementation process under the Maxicap is essentially closed to participation of groups outside of the health care industry. Despite its acknowledged influence in the legislature and the potential impact of higher health care costs on its membership, organized labor has no role in hospital cost containment (Hyde 1993). Similarly, public interest groups are excluded from the process due to the confidential nature of the budget negotiations with individual hospitals. Neither Blue Cross nor HARI have shown any inclination to expand group participation in the hospital rate-setting process in the foreseeable future.

RHODE ISLAND'S APPROACH TO COST CONTAINMENT

State efforts to control health care costs in Rhode Island have been endorsed by health care providers as long as these measures did not pose a significant threat to the administrative autonomy or fiscal health of hospitals. Successful programs have been jointly negotiated and administered by public officials and private groups, and both the state's unique approach to hospital rate-setting and the certificate-of-need process have enjoyed consistent support from both providers and third-party payers. In contrast, where state officials introduced regulatory initiatives without the backing of the hospital industry, recurring tensions undermined the political support necessary to overcome resistance from HARI. Private groups retain an upper hand in policy-making debates in the Ocean State, for the administrative capacity of state agencies remains weak. State officials depend heavily on their private sector counterparts for the information and expertise needed to implement regulatory solutions. As a result, providers and payers have been actively represented in defining policy choices, legislative decision-making, and program implementation. The one exception to this pattern proves the rule, for the state legislature's decision to enact an annual cap on hospital capital expenditures in 1983 marked the beginning of a decade of conflict between HARI and the Department of Health over both the legitimacy and administration of the program. After more than ten years of opposition, hospitals succeeded in their efforts to repeal the limits on capital expenditures in 1994.

Health planning has a long history in Rhode Island, dating back to the mid-1960s; private planning efforts predated the passage of federal and state certificate-of-need legislation. In 1968, Rhode Island became the second state in the nation to regulate hospital capital projects. The legislature's decision to regulate capital construction won the endorsement of the hospital industry and a special legislative commission appointed to study the rapid increase in hospital charges in Rhode Island during the 1960s as a means to control rising costs by limiting the construction of unneeded health care facilities. Despite the inherent risks involved in ceding regulatory authority to the state, hospitals viewed CON as a less onerous alternative to state rate-setting. Blue Cross and Blue Shield of Rhode Island, on the other hand, enthusiastically supported facilities planning as a means to control its costs over the past two decades. In general, providers have favored private planning initiatives that did not threaten their autonomy and opposed planning functions lodged within the Department of Health as unnecessary intrusions on medical practice.

In the first decade of Rhode Island's CON process, one senior vice president at a Brown-affiliated teaching hospital noted that "if an institution put together a superb argument for additional funding for new services or facilities, it had a good chance of outmaneuvering its fellow hospitals." The limitations of Rhode Island's existing CON legislation were readily apparent during the debate over an application from Women & Infants' Hospital to replace its aging facility in the early 1980s. One hospital administrator explained, "no one had ever envisioned the replacement of a hospital, but dropping out of the sky was a $50 million project."[2] The Department's proposal to strengthen the CON process won the endorsement of a special legislative commission to study health care capital expenditures chaired by state Representative Anthony Carceri. In its 1982 report to the General Assembly, the commission argued that the "health care system, like individuals, must be held more closely to the discipline of a budget."

The passage of the Health Care System Affordability Act by both the House (83-0) and the Senate (45-0) in 1984 followed the recommendations of officials in the Department of Health and the final report of the Carceri commission, both of whom argued that certificate-of-need would be more effective if a statewide capital expenditure limit were imposed on new construction projects (Tierney, Waters, and Rosenberg 1982, 181). The legislation established a ceiling on total capital expenditures and required the Health Services Council to review proposals for (1) new facilities in excess of $600,000, (2) increases of ten or more acute-care beds or 10% of existing capacity, (3) the addition of new services which increase operating expenses by $250,000 or more, and (4) the acquisition of health care equipment requiring an expenditure of more than $400,000.[3] All CON applications subject to CONCAP review were reviewed in a single "batch" each year to foster a comparison of each proposal's relative merits. After projects were ranked in order of both affordability and need, applications would be approved in order until the annual CONCAP budget was exhausted.[4] The Health Services Council, however, was not required to fully deplete the CONCAP; each CON approval reduced the amount available for other projects, creating a zero-sum game among applicants. The actual dollar limit of the CONCAP reflected the estimated cost of the annual capital-related operating expenditures, interest, depreciation, and leasehold expenses negotiated during the prospective reimbursement process (Scott et al. 1987). Under the CONCAP process, each certificate-of-need application approved by the state's Health Services Council (HSC) reduced the amount available for other projects; the cost of interest and depreciation for all projects under review was not allowed to exceed the annual negotiated budget.

Rhode Island has more than twenty years of experience with prospective reimbursement for hospital care, making it one of the nation's longest running health care cost-containment programs. The enabling legislation governing hospital reimbursement passed the legislature with little debate in 1971 and has been amended only twice, once in 1984 when new limitations on the construction of capital projects were inserted, and later in 1994 when the limits were removed from the overall budget negotiation process. Since 1974, state officials, provider groups, and third-party payers have jointly administered a global expenditure cap for hospital services (the Maxicap) with a modest commitment of staff and resources. Representatives from the Hospital Association of Rhode Island, Blue Cross, and the state meet in March or April of each year to negotiate a global operating budget.

The Maxicap itself is not a binding ceiling but rather serves as a target for aggregate statewide hospital expenses over the next fiscal year once allowances for new programs have been taken into account. Blue Cross and HARI each appoint negotiating teams of four or five members to represent their positions. While the state budget officer is included in the negotiations, the team from Blue Cross typically acts on behalf of the state since both parties share a common goal of controlling costs. Negotiations revolve around estimates of projected increases in the cost of various inputs such as salaries, fringe benefits, depreciation and interest expenses, and supplies (Leco 1976).[5] The sum of all expenditure categories plus allowance for capital costs associated with new programs and facilities represent the negotiated Maxicap for the upcoming fiscal year.

After the Maxicap has been negotiated by representatives of the hospital association and Blue Cross, the focus of the process shifts to the proposed budgets of individual hospitals for the next fiscal year (Leco 1976). While the overall Maxicap sets a target for statewide hospital expenditure growth, the increases of individual hospitals often vary considerably under the program. This flexibility allows budget negotiations to accommodate the needs of individual institutions while controlling systemwide costs. For example, a hospital confronted with unusual demands in a particular year may receive an above-average increase in its budget, while other institutions receive smaller increases. Although the results of individual negotiations are allowed to vary, the total increase in expenditures for all hospitals may not exceed the Maxicap's negotiated ceiling for that year.

The Maxicap process, however, is self-enforced; no penalties are meted out for hospitals that exceed their budgets.[6] Furthermore, no enforcement mechanism exists to ensure that overall hospital expenditures fall within the negotiated Maxicap. The informal nature of the process reflects the realities of policy-making under a negotiated regime, for a binding expenditure cap creates a zero-sum game for hospitals that pits institutions against each other. The consultative nature of the Maxicap negotiations has won praise from both public and private participants and has bolstered the legitimacy of the rate-setting process in the eyes of providers. In the absence of consensus among participating groups, negotiated regimes are ill-equipped to deal with redistributive issues.

The emphasis on mutual accommodation within the Maxicap process is also evident once a statewide expenditure target has been established. After individual hospitals file their proposed annual budget with the Department of Business Regulation, budget negotiations continue between Blue Cross and individual hospitals until a contract is signed, a process which can last several months. If the negotiating teams from Blue Cross and the hospital remain deadlocked after exchanging "last best offers," the Maxicap guidelines call for the appointment of an impartial mediator to facilitate an agreement.[7] Failure to resolve contractual disagreements through mediation subjects both parties to binding arbitration. Arbitration, however, is an undesirable option, for the arbitrator has only two choices—he or she must choose one of the last best offers, but not any point in between. The legislature's directive that the parties employ the services of mediators and/or an arbitrator to forge a mutually acceptable agreement illustrates a defining principle of negotiated regimes: mutual adjustment among stakeholders. Unlike case-based or per diem systems, decisions concerning the level of reimbursement must be agreed to by all parties; the state lacks the authority to impose a settlement that is unacceptable to the principal stakeholders.

Negotiations during the Maxicap process also determine utilization targets for ancillary services (e.g., radiology, laboratory, diagnostic imaging, outpatient surgery). Fluctuations in a hospital's projected patient volume of 3% or more activate a series of adjustments, known as volume corridors, to reflect the effects of these changes.[8] Increases in volume are covered by so-called "upside" corridors, which are designed to reflect changes in the marginal cost of providing care to additional patients. Upside corridors reimburse hospitals only for the additional labor costs that they incur by adding personnel to cope with a greater number of patients and do not provide for fixed costs associated with capital requirements or facilities. Similarly, when volume declines, hospitals must maintain essential services such as pediatrics, obstetrics, and intensive-care units despite a reduced patient load. During the 1980s, "downside" corridors insulated Rhode Island hospitals from sharp declines in inpatient revenues which accompanied the introduction of Medicare's prospective payment system and the industrywide trend toward a shorter average length of stay.

A negotiated regime is based upon consensual decision-making and bargaining among participating groups and institutions. The Maxicap process relies upon the voluntary compliance of member hospitals, who continue to support the system despite fundamental shifts in the pattern of inpatient care during the 1980s. In particular, the retention of volume corridors reflected the interests of hospitals in maintaining a stable revenue stream in the face of falling inpatient utilization. Even if the state and Blue Cross had wanted to abandon the system of volume corridors, it is unlikely that they could have done so without cooperation from the state's hospitals since any change to the Maxicap's reimbursement process required the approval of each of the participating organizations. Since neither volume corridors nor the Maxicap were included in the enabling legislation that created the state's prospective payment system, both were "contractual issues" subject to negotiation between individual payers and providers.

Rhode Island's decision to seek a Section 1115 waiver from the Health Care Financing Administration (HCFA) to enroll all AFDC-eligible women and children in managed care programs continues to receive broad-based support from physicians, hospitals, and third-party payers (Freyer 1996). At the end of its first year, more than 58,000 Medicaid recipients had been enrolled in four managed care providers under contract to the state through the RIte Care program administered by the Department of Human Services. Due to a slow initial enrollment process hampered by delays in licensing Neighborhood Health Plan, the state's first Medicaid-only HMO formed by a network of community health centers, many participating health centers lost patients and revenues during the first year (Demkovich 1996f). By 1996, enrollment in RIte Care had risen to more than 70,000, including more than 3,000 previously uninsured women and children (HCFA 1996d).

State officials actively solicited input from providers, payers, and consumer advocates during both the application and implementation process in 1993-94. As a result, Rhode Island's managed care waiver enjoyed strong support from the key participants in the state's health care policy-issue network, including Brown University's School of Medicine, Blue Cross, all participating HMOs, the local chapter of the American Academy of Pediatrics, and the Rhode Island Medical Society (State of Rhode Island 1993). The consultative approach to decision-making resembled the process which created the Maxicap, as the state enlisted the support of private actors to achieve its goal of controlling costs and improving access to health services for the uninsured. The state's embrace of managed care as a means of controlling Medicaid costs, however, did not signal a move away from negotiated expenditure limits. Instead, hospital executives publicly reaffirmed their support for the Maxicap process and touted the findings of a report by KPMG Peat Marwick (1996) which cited the state's hospitals as the most "cost effective" in the nation (Read 1996).

Although its unique approach to health care regulation has not received the national attention accorded programs in New Jersey and other states, Rhode Island has been cited as one of the six most successful prospective payment systems in the nation (Coelen et al. 1988). Early discussions of Rhode Island's experience with prospective reimbursement in the 1970s suggested that prospective rate-setting that relied upon a review of hospital budgets by state officials did not have a statistically significant impact on cost inflation. Based on a review of the state's experience with rate-setting from 1971 to 72, Hellinger (1976) contended that the budget review process was "inherently cumbersome" due to the complex nature of the budget negotiations (see Table 5.1). While these findings were disputed by Zimmerman, Buechner, and Thornberry (1977), Rhode Island's distinctive approach to regulating hospital reimbursement fell into disfavor among federal officials and never became a national model for regulatory reform. Nevertheless, Rhode Island's rate of hospital inflation was below the national average for ten of the first fourteen years of the program's operation (Levit et al. 1993). As with many regulatory programs, the performance of Rhode Island's global-budgeting approach also improved over time, and compares favorably with other states that employed formula-based (e.g., per-case or per diem) rate-setting systems (see Table 5.2).

A review of Rhode Island's experience with a reformed CON process reveals that the state has successfully controlled capital-related costs over the past decade. Since the introduction of the CONCAP, Rhode Island's approval rate dropped considerably, from 76.2% in the years preceding its adoption to 64.5% during the ten-year period from 1984 to 1993 (Hackey and Fuller 1995). From 1984 to 1993, the state's CON program had the lowest approval rate among the New England states. Passage of the CONCAP legislation reduced interest expenses by requiring hospitals to increase their equity participation, or "down payment," on new capital projects (Donahue et al. 1992). A higher percentage of equity funding for capital projects, in turn, constrained overall hospital-related health care costs by reducing institutional expenditures associated with servicing capital debts. The results of Rhode Island's ten-year experiment with a reformed CON process are clear: capital-related costs for Rhode Island's eleven acute-care hospitals fell

---

TABLE 5.1   An Overview of Rhode Island's Maxicap Negotiations

Stage 1	Review of Proposals by the "Committee of Eight" ⇓
Stage 2	Maxicap Negotiations ———— Mediation/Arbitration ⇓
Stage 3	Hospital Budget Submissions ⇓
Stage 4	Budget Review and Analysis ⇓
Stage 5	Budget Negotiations with Individual Hospitals ——— Mediation/Arbitration ⇓
Stage 6	Prospective Rate Determination ⇓
Stage 7	Year End Adjustments for Volume and Major Contingencies ⇓
Stage 8	Year End Settlement ⇓
Stage 9	Final Adjusted Maxicap

---

well below national and regional averages (Hackey and Fuller 1995). The median capital-expense ratio for Rhode Island's eleven acute-care hospitals (0.05) was the lowest in the region and the second lowest in the United States in 1992 (Cleverly 1993, 93), indicating that the state's hospitals had an unusually low level of debt relative to their counterparts in other states.[9]

The utilization rate of health care facilities also provides insights into the effectiveness of state CON controls. Despite growing competition in the state's health insurance marketplace and a national trend toward lower utilization of inpatient services, the median occupancy rate for acute-care hospitals in Rhode Island exceeded both the regional and national medians. The state's median occupancy rate of 68.9% was the fifth highest rate in the nation in 1993. Rhode Island did not experience a surge in the construction of ambulatory surgical centers, freestanding imaging centers, or new hospital facilities following the termination of federal planning programs in 1987. Since the state's

TABLE 5.2 Percentage Change in Total Expenditures by Community Hospitals, 1974 to 1992

State	1974–80	1981–87	1988–92
Maryland	133.5	56.6	41.9
Massachusetts	105.9	56.1	39.2
New Jersey	114.3	74.1	64.3
New York	82.2	64.9	48.4
Rhode Island	104.5	68.9	37.9
U.S. average	135.6	69.4	47.0

Source: American Hospital Association, *Hospital Statistics*, various years.

hospital bed capacity was not "overbuilt," decreasing lengths of stay and changing treatment patterns (e.g., from inpatient to outpatient surgery) had a more moderate impact on hospitals in Rhode Island than elsewhere.

The effect of an aggregate cap on capital expenditures is particularly evident in the aging of hospitals' physical plant during the 1980s. The median age of the state's acute-care hospitals (9.51 years) was considerably higher than the national median and the median of all other states in the region except Connecticut. In 1992, the average age of the fixed assets of hospitals in Rhode Island was the third highest in the nation (Cleverly 1993). Since hospitals in Rhode Island were often unable to add new services or construct new facilities even when they had demonstrated "need," the CONCAP also encouraged the development of collaborative approaches for imaging and cardiac services. To meet demand for new technologies in a cost-effective manner, the Department of Health issued several requests for proposals in the late 1980s to encourage long-range planning. In the case of magnetic resonance imaging (MRI), a statewide nonprofit MRI network emerged as the solution to the need for the cost-effective diffusion of imaging services. Participating hospitals agreed to share MRI technology through a mobile network which provided MRI units for each institution at least two days per week. Furthermore, since radiologists employed by the MRI network performed and analyzed tests at each hospital, individual institutions were spared the cost of building and staffing permanent facilities (Hackey and Fuller 1995).

Rhode Island's experience demonstrates the effectiveness of a budget cap for controlling hospital capital expenditures. In particular, the CONCAP severely limited opportunities to "outmaneuver" the CON process after its introduction in 1984. Unlike an open-ended CON process in which an unlimited number of projects could be approved if they demonstrated "need," the CONCAP's emphasis on statewide affordability created a zero-sum game for providers. A ceiling on capital costs forces decision makers to prioritize programs and choose those projects that are the most cost effective (Young 1991). The very stringency of the process, however, ultimately proved to be its undoing, for the CONCAP was repealed by the General Assembly at the request of the governor's office on its tenth anniversary in 1994. Under a negotiated regime, policies that challenge the prerogatives and autonomy of major stakeholders become lightning rods for disaffected groups and may lose their legitimacy. Elected officials, for their part, are frequently tempted to back away from contested initiatives in order to preserve support for other activities.

THE NATURE OF THE DECISION-MAKING PROCESS IN RHODE ISLAND

The small scale of the health care policy-issue network in Rhode Island is particularly suited to meso-corporatist bargaining, for each of the participants in the state's prospective reimbursement system is empowered to bargain on behalf of its members. Aside from the immediate participants, few people in either state government or the private sector are even aware of the negotiations that occur each spring. Consumer groups, proponents of universal health care, and advocates for the poor are present in the Ocean State, but none has pressed for the right to participate in the process. Indeed, since negotiations over Blue Cross' contracts with individual hospitals occur within the Maxicap negotiations, it is doubtful that new groups would be allowed to participate. The health care policy-issue network in Rhode Island is neither diverse nor dense. Since representatives from the state medical society (or one of its professional associations), HARI and its members, and the state's third-party health insurers are involved in developing most health-related legislation, many differences among participants are resolved before they arrive at the legislature. Furthermore, "because of the state's small size and its structure of overlapping elites, political bargaining is done mostly on a face-to-face basis by people who know one another well" (Hyde 1993, 310).

The formal incorporation of interest groups in setting the Maxicap and negotiating individual hospital budgets is best described as a system of "administrative corporatism."[10] Corporatist policy-making is commonplace in negotiated regimes, for bargaining among public and private elites in the decision-making process and the formal delegation of administrative tasks to private trade associations is consistent with the principle of consultation and mutual adjustment that governs such regimes. Rhode Island's prospective reimbursement system offers a clear example of corporatist-interest intermediation at the state level. Although Wilson (1982) and others (Salisbury 1979) have detailed many reasons for the lack of corporatism in the United States, the emergence of administrative corporatism in Rhode Island is understandable in the context of the state's weak political institutions. Unable to convince legislators or the governor to support new grants of regulatory authority, state officials brokered a compromise with payers and providers to achieve their ends.

The pattern of mutual accommodation between the state and private interests is most evident in the negotiation of individual hospital budgets under the Maxicap. The lack of specificity in the state's prospective reimbursement process limited the development of new institutional capacity to monitor and manage the payment system, which has largely been delegated to representatives from Blue Cross and HARI. Regulatory programs administered by or in partnership with representatives from the regulated industry are ill-equipped to impose penalties on member institutions, for to do so invites fragmentation and conflict among constituent organizations. Rhode Island's experience is consistent with this pattern, for the Maxicap process permits hospitals to petition for exceptions to their budgets for disasters and other "major contingencies" such as new labor agreements, rising malpractice costs, and costs associated with the state's MRI network. Furthermore, negotiators from Blue Cross and the hospital association have frequently accommodated the unique circumstances or needs of individual hospitals in a particular year.

The corporatist underpinnings of the Maxicap process can be traced to its inception in the early 1970s. The Maxicap emerged in response to a perceived "cost crisis" in hospital room rates; by 1966, the General Assembly created a fourteen-member commission (known as the Brosco Commission) to study the feasibility of a state rate-setting system for Rhode Island. By the end of the decade, however, the system of retrospective reimbursement based on "usual, customary, and reasonable" patient charges came under fire amid growing concerns about health care inflation. Although the Brosco Commission's final report to the legislature noted that "there is a clamor for government to do something about rising hospital costs and charges," it offered few solutions and refused to endorse a regulatory strategy to control hospital costs. Indeed, the commission asserted that "the issue at this time is not one of arbitrary regulation of hospital rates" (Brosco Commission 1967, 48).

Hospital cost inflation continued unabated in the years following the commission's report. Several years of double-digit increases in Blue Cross premiums drew renewed interest in controlling hospital costs, as rising costs received considerable attention from the media in the late 1960s. After a series of explosive rate hearings in 1969, the Rhode Island Department of Business Regulation (DBR) urged Blue Cross to contemplate fundamental reforms to control health care costs. State officials, however, did not seek to impose a solution on the industry through legislation or rule-making, but instead enlisted the help of private payers and providers to forge a solution.

Throughout 1969 and 1970, officials from Blue Cross and the Hospital Association of Rhode Island initiated discussions aimed at changing the system from retrospective cost-based reimbursement to a prospective-payment model. Against this backdrop, Larry Hill, a vice president at Rhode Island Hospital (the state's largest), suggested that individual hospitals might negotiate their budgets with payers. Together, representatives from HARI, Blue Cross, and Rhode Island Hospital developed a model to govern negotiations between Rhode Island Hospital and Blue Cross for the hospital's FY1971 budget. Before the hospital's fiscal year began in September, the three parties successfully negotiated a budget agreement, proving that the strategy was workable. Even though the agreement was negotiated in private, with no direct involvement by the state, the savings were substantial; the final settlement reduced the hospital's budget by more than one million dollars.

Public rate hearings over the Blue Cross-proposed premium increases for FY1971 were held throughout the negotiations over Rhode Island Hospital's budget. HARI had planned to learn from Rhode Island Hospital's experience and incorporate it into the budget cycles of other hospitals at a later date. However, the prospect of another round of confrontational rate hearings before the DBR put pressure on the association to realize significant cost savings or face the threat of more extensive state regulation in the near future. HARI's membership agreed to the basic framework of the new program, enabling the hospitals to negotiate their budgets with Blue Cross for FY1972 and beyond.

The new system emerged as a result of extensive consultation between Blue Cross and the state's hospitals; once private negotiations concluded, state officials simply ratified the existing consensus as policy. Together, Blue Cross and the hospital association took the proposed plan to the director of the state's Department of Business Regulation, who, in the words of one HARI official, "basically blessed the proposal to move off cost reimbursement as a retrospective system and to move onto a system of negotiated budgets." This agreement was formalized by the legislature in an amendment to the original statute governing Blue Cross reimbursement in 1971 (Chapter 206 of the Public Laws of 1971). The amendment required all hospitals to enter into budget negotiations with Blue Cross and the state's budget officer at least ninety days prior to the start of the fiscal year. In addition, the legislation required that hospitals and third-party payers (e.g., Blue Cross and the state budget officer) reach an agreement over operating budgets and "related statistics" no later than thirty days prior to the beginning of each fiscal year.

The enabling legislation merely outlined the process of negotiation and left the fundamental issues raised by rate-setting (e.g., the form of reimbursement) up to the parties that had drafted the bill. The meso-corporatist nature of the new regulatory process was apparent in the partnership between state officials and representatives from hospitals and Blue Cross. The state budget officer served a dual role in the process as a purchaser of care and as a public representative. In effect, Rhode Island's new prospective reimbursement process delegated implementation of the system to private groups with participation by the state. Unlike Maryland and New York, which embarked on rate-setting by creating specialized bureaucratic agencies to oversee the regulation of hospital expenditures in the early 1970s, legislators conferred no new powers on the Department of Health, nor did they seriously constrain provider autonomy.

Rhode Island's experiment with negotiated hospital budgets had an inauspicious beginning. As talks were about to begin, President Nixon's Economic Stabilization Program imposed a national freeze on wage and price increases. The proposed prospective reimbursement process was incompatible with the Nixon administration's system of wage and price controls, for the negotiations between state officials, Blue Cross, and the hospitals centered around total operating budgets, not unit prices.[11] The hospitals participated as planned during the first year of the new program by guaranteeing their budgets in the system, creating a base for the first round of negotiations that was set to begin for the FY1972 budgets. How they would achieve this goal in the context of the price freeze was unclear; negotiations for FY1972 were suspended indefinitely. Faced with conflicting state and federal mandates, a global operating budget for all hospitals was proposed as a solution to the hospitals' dilemma. As one HARI official present at the time recalled,

> The governor's office asked if the [federal] Price Commission would [allow] us to negotiate our own ceiling . . . and let us decide how to distribute it. . . . If we could do it ourselves, some hospitals might get more and others might get less, but we could do it [based] on an average. We came

up with the idea of a Maxicap which would be an aggregate limit on the expenses of all of the participating hospitals . . . that enabled us to get a waiver from the Price Commission to let us do our own control program and negotiate the budgets.

In the process of pursuing a waiver from the Price Commission, Rhode Island's proposal caught the eye of federal officials in the Department of Health, Education and Welfare (HEW). Using their new authority under the 1972 Social Security Amendments, Medicare officials offered Rhode Island a waiver from HEW's traditional cost-based principles of reimbursement for FY1975. Even though the Economic Stabilization Program ceased operations in June 1974, Medicare officials expressed an interest in continuing the state's unique experiment for a three-year period. Medicare's participation in the new system brought Rhode Island close to having an all-payer rate-setting system; from 1975 to 1977, roughly 85% of all payers in Rhode Island were covered under the state's prospective rate negotiation program.[12]

From the beginning, however, HEW officials did express concern about the corporatist nature of the experiment. As one HARI official noted, "At the end of 1976 we had all sorts of struggles with Medicare. They didn't like the idea of negotiating—they were more of the opinion that they'd tell you how to do things than in our system, where you never got exactly what you wanted, but neither did they." However, since hospitals were legally required to engage in annual budget negotiations, the Maxicap process continued with only minor modifications between Blue Cross, Medicaid, and the industry representatives after the end of the federal waiver in 1977.

More than two decades after its introduction, Rhode Island's prospective payment system still enjoys enthusiastic support from key interest groups. In the words of one senior hospital executive, the process "may not be perfect, but it's ultimately stronger than it is weak and it works—that's why there haven't been any specific changes in it." This diffuse support (Easton 1975) is invaluable to the long-term programmatic success of Rhode Island's cost-containment strategy. The active participation of providers and payers in setting the Maxicap and negotiating individual hospital budgets lends legitimacy to the process; while sporadic conflicts have occurred between Blue Cross and individual hospitals, no institution has challenged the legality of the process or questioned the goals of the state's reimbursement methodology. Continued support for the Maxicap is also a by-product of the stability of the health care policy-issue network in Rhode Island. Since no significant shifts in the relative influence of providers and purchasers of care occurred during the past two decades, participants have had few incentives to radically alter a process which serves their needs.

Rhode Island's negotiated policy regime, however, differs sharply from that of other states in its emphasis on mutual accommodation rather than state controls to regulate systemwide costs. One reason for the system's stability is the continuity in personnel involved in the negotiations. The Maxicap process is small in scale and highly personalized, and participants have generally worked together for years. The principal negotiators in the early 1990s, Jack Grant and Armand Leco for Blue Cross, and William Sweeney for HARI, were instrumental in creating the program two decades earlier.

In addition, since the essential elements of the state's regulatory system were hammered out in private negotiations between Blue Cross and the hospitals, the system continued to enjoy support from both hospitals and third-party payers. As one senior HARI official noted in 1990, "Our hospitals have taken pride in participating in what we would argue is essentially a voluntary or quasi-voluntary system." While individual institutions and players may be dissatisfied with the results of negotiations in a given year, key stakeholders continue to express confidence that the system works fairly and achieves its goal of controlling costs (Urcioli 1996).

HEALTH CARE POLICY-MAKING IN A NEGOTIATED REGIME

Negotiated regimes are characterized by a high degree of interdependence among public and private groups within an issue network. All participants must cooperate in order to achieve their goals or objectives, for unilateral action is unlikely to be successful in a policy-making environment dominated by active peak associations with competing interests. In the absence of consultation, the end result of legislative bargaining is often stalemate; fissures among private advocacy coalitions prevent either side from prevailing on important issues at the expense of others. The state, for its part, lacks both the statutory authority and administrative capacity to enforce its preferences on private groups. This pattern of policy-making is particularly evident in Rhode Island, where both Blue Cross and the hospital industry have enjoyed strong support from legislators in recent decades. Proposals viewed as a threat by one of the principal stakeholders in the system have fared poorly in the legislature, which has encouraged the resolution of group differences through private bargaining.

Even if they were predisposed to do so, state policymakers in Rhode Island were ill-equipped to assume a leadership role on health care financing issues over the past two decades. Elected officials in Rhode Island have a difficult time in overcoming the state's reputation for political corruption and "honest graft." At the turn of the century, muckraking journalist Lincoln Steffens described Rhode Island as a "state for sale"; decades later, Neal Peirce observed that "the apparent waning of outright corruption [did] not mean that the old political patronage system [was] dead in Rhode Island" in the 1970s (Peirce 1976, 164). The state's political institutions and public officials have been rocked by allegations of scandal and impropriety in recent years. The collapse of the Rhode Island Savings and Deposit Insurance Corporation (RISDIC) in 1991 led to the closure of numerous banks and credit unions statewide and threw the state into an economic tailspin (see Cornwell 1992). A series of televised hearings and the hiring of special prosecutors revealed that legislative oversight of RISDIC, a state-chartered private insurer, had been sporadic. The RISDIC scandal, the indictment of former governor Edward DiPrete, and the resignation of the sitting chief justice of the state's Supreme Court confirmed that the "incestuous" character of policy-making in Rhode Island continued in the 1990s.

The RISDIC crisis provided a number of important lessons for health care policy-making in the Ocean State, for the state's banking fiasco highlighted the inability of legislators to practice effective oversight of the regulated industry. A part-time legislature dominated by the Democratic Party was ill-equipped to develop and monitor complex regulatory policies, so in both banking and health care, private interests were granted substantial autonomy to wield public authority through quasi-public negotiations and administrative arrangements. The limitations of the state's policy-making institutions and the accommodative nature of the decision-making and implementation process is evident from the inception of Rhode Island's rate-setting and certificate-of-need programs in the late 1960s.

The basic outlines of the Maxicap process were hammered out in private negotiations between representatives from Blue Cross and HARI in 1970; since the details of the state's prospective reimbursement system were not spelled out in legislation, the statutory powers granted to state officials were quite weak. While the legislature mandated negotiations between state officials, Blue Cross, and hospitals, the enabling legislation did not specify ground rules to guide the negotiations. State officials do not possess the authority to mete out penalties to noncompliant institutions, and the Maxicap itself lacks an enforcement mechanism. Furthermore, since the enabling legislation did not specify the nature of the state's reimbursement methodology (e.g., per diem or case-based), the state's bargaining position in the negotiations is intimately linked to the goals of Blue Cross in the reimbursement negotiations. As a result of the legislature's decision to ratify the private agreement negotiated by Blue Cross and HARI, administration of the prospective reimbursement system remains in the hands of the principal private stakeholders. While the collaborative nature of the Maxicap process limits the ability of state officials to control costs without the acquiescence of health providers, the collaborative nature of the administrative process is a political asset that has insulated the program from provider opposition.

The CONCAP process offers a useful contrast to this model of mutual accommodation, for hospitals never supported an aggregate ceiling on capital expenditures and lobbied against the program from its inception. The passage of the CONCAP was an exception to the typical pattern of legislative policy-making in Rhode Island, for legislators uncharacteristically endorsed the recommendations of a study commission chaired by a well respected member of the House of Representatives, Representative Anthony Carceri. As a member of the state Health Services Council, Carceri persuaded his colleagues that the state's CON process needed to be strengthened in order to control costs. While legislators deferred to the recommendations of their experienced colleague in 1984, once the CONCAP was implemented it immediately drew fire from providers. Over time, as the program's legislative sponsors and supporters left state government, the conflict-ridden process became increasingly vulnerable; with few supporters and many influential detractors, the CONCAP succumbed to provider opposition in 1994.

In the absence of a previously negotiated agreement among payers and providers, state officials have been largely unsuccessful in their efforts to increase the capacity of state policy-making institutions, particularly those lodged within the Department of Health. After the expiration of federal health planning requirements in 1986, HARI and its members successfully lobbied legislators to defeat the Department of Health's proposal to create a new state-funded state health services coordinating council (SHCC) to preserve the state's health planning efforts. More recently, proposals to create an integrated trauma system among the state's acute-care hospitals were met by fierce opposition from hospitals, who refused to cede authority over the designation and certification of trauma centers to the Department of Health. In both cases, providers supported the creation of quasi-public planning bodies with broad representation from hospitals, physicians, and third-party payers in lieu of state action.

State officials have adopted a "hands off" approach to health care regulation, for most policy initiatives originate with providers or payers. Public officials, however, regularly enlist the aid of Blue Cross, HARI, and the Rhode Island Medical Society to lobby for issues in the package of legislative proposals submitted with the governor's annual budget message. Few issue entrepreneurs have emerged in the past two decades to press for fundamental changes in the state's health care financing system. On more than one occasion over the past decade, state officials formed "blue ribbon commissions" to explore the challenges facing the health care system, but none of these efforts was adopted as a blueprint for systemic reform by legislative leaders or the governor's office.

The prominent role of health care providers and third-party payers in formulating and implementing policy in Rhode Island is a consequence of the limited capacity of state political institutions. State revenues have lagged behind expenditures in recent years, creating a serious structural deficit for policymakers. In an effort to improve the state's business climate, public officials have resisted proposals to raise sales or income taxes and instead have sought to downsize the state work force through attrition and cut existing programs. Existing state institutions are ill-equipped to undertake a leadership role in comprehensive health care reform. The legislature, for its part, remains underpaid and woefully understaffed despite a recent pay increase for members approved by voters in 1994. The governor's office sets the legislative agenda each year by forwarding a list of departmental priorities to the General Assembly, but departments frequently must advocate for their own legislative priorities with little support from the governor's policy staff. At the cabinet level, the capacity of state departments varies widely; some departments have acquired a strong professional orientation, while others continue to lack the expertise or staffing to effectively challenge private interests involved in health care policy-making.

The Legislature

Despite Republican successes in other statewide contests during the 1980s, the legislature remains a bastion of Democratic power. Democrats have held more than 70% of the seats in the House in every year since 1972. In the Senate, Republicans reached a high water mark in 1982, when they won 21 out of 50 seats; in most years, however, sizable Democratic majorities in both houses were sufficient to override gubernatorial vetoes. In 1996, Democrats remained in a comfortable position, as the party controlled 40 of 50 seats in the Senate and 84 of 100 seats in the House. Policy-making in the legislature has been tightly controlled by the leadership of the Democratic majority for several decades. Nearly four decades ago, Duane Lockard (1956, 212) observed that "members of the General Assembly may at times upset the plans of the leadership, but in the vast majority of the cases the final word rests with the leaders." Little has changed in the intervening years, despite a series of procedural reforms intended to limit the ability of the leadership to quash bills and to encourage consultation with individual members.[13] In each chamber, committee assignments, access to the legislative calendar, and office space rest squarely in the hands of the Speaker of the House and the Senate majority leader and their allies. Building seniority within the legislature is not a difficult proposition, for the weakness of the state's Republican Party and the lack of a viable "reform coalition" within the Democratic Party ensures that many legislative leaders are unopposed in both primaries and general elections.

As a result of their weak position, Republicans in both the House and the Senate have been limited to a strategy of "inconsequential opposition" (Jones 1968) on most significant policy issues. In recent years, however, rival Democratic factions in both chambers limited the control of legislative leaders over rank-and-file members. The legislative leadership has been widely criticized for persistent infighting over office space and other perks among rival factions of Democratic senators and for reports of personal improprieties among prominent members of the House and the Senate. Disputes among factions within the Democratic Party, however, seldom offered Republicans an opportunity to influence the outcome of legislation.

Rhode Island voters approved a sweeping reform package aimed at improving the professionalism and ethical climate within the General Assembly in 1994. Salaries for members were increased from five dollars per day to $10,000 per year, and legislators' ability to grant themselves lucrative state pensions for their legislative service was sharply restricted (Cornwell and Moakley 1996). Beginning in the year 2000, the size of the House will be reduced from 100 members to 75, while the Senate will fall to 38 from 50. Professionalism remains a problem, for despite the recent pay increase, most members are employed full-time outside of the General Assembly. Even experienced legislators often lack policy expertise, for members have few staff to conduct independent research into policy problems. In 1994, the ratio of legislators to staff members in the Senate was 8:1, while the ratio of members of the House of Representatives to staff was 7:1 (Council of State Governments 1994, 154).

Party discipline in the General Assembly remained high in the 1990s; private negotiations between the leadership and affected parties resolve most differences before they reach the floor. Legislators also regard lobbyists as a vital source of information about the policy implications of legislation before the General Assembly. Two legislators summed up the importance of interest groups in the policy-making process in Rhode Island when they observed that "'lobbyists are the most valuable resource we have' and '[There is] no greater service for a legislator than having a group of well-informed lobbyists'" (quoted in Hyde 1993, 310). In recognition of this, the state has not seriously considered lobbying reforms to limit the amount or timing of lobbyists' campaign contributions or prohibit "contingent compensation" of professional lobbyists (Council of State Governments 1994, 490).

In addition, structural barriers limit the ability of the General Assembly to serve as either an incubator of innovative policy options or as an effective oversight body. The short legislative session of sixty days seriously restricts legislative debate over many issues and hinders the ability of members to engage in meaningful oversight activities when the legislature is not in session. Passage of the budget, however, remains the principal goal for both the Senate and the House during extended sessions, as members quickly adjourn once their required duties have been met. Leadership in both chambers have also come under fire from junior legislators and the press for their habit of ramming legislation through in the wee hours of the morning during the closing days of the legislative session. Members often complained that they were not even sure of the contents of the bills they voted for, let alone the relative merits of various policy proposals (McVicar 1996).

Members also lack full-time secretarial support, and aside from the party leadership in each house, most members do not have an office at the state capitol building. The committee structure of the General Assembly also lacks specialization. The Senate and the House each have six standing committees; six joint committees have members from both houses. With the exception of the finance committees in both houses and the legislative leadership, most committees also lack dedicated policy staff. In contrast, the leadership in both houses has added staff in recent years as a means to centralize control over the legislative agenda (Cornwell and Moakley 1996); by 1996, the House Finance Committee employed eight policy analysts, including the former director of the state budget office. The legislature has traditionally held the upper hand in its relationship with the governor's office, for the formal powers of the governorship in Rhode Island are among the weakest in the nation (Beyle 1990). The influence of legislative leaders has been particularly evident since 1990; budget and policy proposals of both Democrat Bruce Sundlun and his Republican successor, Lincoln Almond, were routinely declared "dead on arrival" by ranking Senators and Representatives. At the behest of the Democratic leadership, legislators also overrode a number of high-profile gubernatorial vetoes, confirming their position as the first among equals in state policymaking circles. The influence of the governor's office reached a low ebb in 1996, when the General Assembly's Democratic leadership overrode Governor Almond's veto of the state budget to end its legislative session.

Bureaucratic Expertise

The administrative capacity of state agencies has fluctuated in Rhode Island in response to changes in the state's fiscal condition. In addition, while the state has competed successfully for a number of federal "capacity-building" grants to improve planning activities over the past two decades, the state has been unwilling to sustain or expand federally sponsored initiatives in the absence of intergovernmental aid. The two principal policy-making agencies on health care issues in Rhode Island are the Department of Human Services, which oversees the Medicaid program and the Maxicap negotiations, and the Department of Health, which manages the state's certificate-of-need process. The DHS inherited responsibility for managing the Maxicap process from the State Budget Office in 1986. The Maxicap continues to be managed through an informal process within DHS; no full-time staff are assigned to hospital negotiations, although the budget negotiations consume a sizable portion of the time of the chief of the department's Division of Medical Services each spring. The approval of Rhode Island's Medicaid managed care waiver led to significant capacity-building effort within the Department of Human Services in 1993 and 1994. Prior to the mid-1990s, DHS had a poor reputation within state government as a department that was overworked and understaffed, and which had few professionally trained policy analysts; the department was the last in the nation to computerize its Medicaid billing services in the early 1990s.

The Department of Health, in contrast, used federal health planning funds to augment its policy-making and planning capacities in the 1970s and 1980s. In stark contrast to the informal arrangements governing prospective reimbursement in Rhode Island, the Department of Health successfully institutionalized its commitment to health planning and certificate-of-need regulation during the 1970s and 1980s. During the early 1970s, Rhode Island's fledgling health planning and capital expenditure efforts received a significant boost as a result of an amendment to the federal Health Planning and Resource Development Act (Pub. L. 93-641). Sponsored by Senator Claiborne Pell (D-RI), it exempted Rhode Island from establishing local citizen planning boards, known as Health Systems Agencies (HSAs). Funds that were channeled to local HSAs in other states were allocated to the Department of Health in Rhode Island, generating a windfall to support the Department of Health's nascent planning activities. In addition to infusing the Department of Health with additional resources, Senator Pell's amendment to Pub. L. 93-641 spared the state the heated conflicts over representation on local HSAs that plagued federally sponsored planning programs elsewhere (Morone 1990a). The centralization of regulatory and planning resources within the Department of Health also prevented the extraordinary fragmentation of decision-making authority over capital expenditure review common in other states (Brown 1981).

During the 1970s and 1980s, the Department of Health recruited and retained a core group of talented administrators and analysts to manage the state's health planning and CON programs. By the mid-1980s, the cadre of health planners that had developed the state's health plans in the 1970s had been promoted to leadership roles. As a result, a strong commitment to planning permeated the department and defined its organizational culture. All of the members of the department's senior management team involved in regulating health care providers in the 1990s (with the exception of the director, who by law must be a physician) had ten or more years of experience with planning and CON. Furthermore, by the late 1980s, the membership of the state Health Services Council, the advisory board that reviewed CON applications, included several former legislators, hospital executives, and business leaders with more than ten years of regulatory experience.

By the mid-1980s, Rhode Island was also a national leader in the creation of statewide health databases; staff at the Department of Health regularly published in professional journals and regularly published policy briefings on the fiscal health of the state's hospitals, health status, and minority health issues. After the expiration of federal health planning subsidies, however, state support for health planning and regulation steadily diminished in the late 1980s and early 1990s. Budget cuts precipitated by the state's emerging fiscal crisis in 1990 and 1991 led to layoffs and furloughs, and demoralized those who remained. The cadre of health policy analysts and planners hired in the 1970s left the department or entered senior administrative positions. Few were replaced in the tight fiscal climate of the 1990s, effectively crippling the department's ability to engage in proactive planning and policy research.

This strategy of gradual attrition, however, contributed to a steady decline in both employee morale and administrative capacity, as the department's authorized level of full-time equivalent positions (FTEs) fell from 475 FTEs in FY1994 to 402 in the governor's FY1997 budget. Overall, state employment (excluding college and university personnel) fell 10.1% from 1985 to 1995; within the Department of Health, state expenditures for "central management" (which includes health planning and health statistics) fell from $2.77 million in FY1991 to $2.11 million in FY1996. Expenditures for health policy and planning also declined sharply in the mid-1990s, from more than $1.9 million in FY1994 to less than $1.2 million in the governor's FY1997 budget. As budgets tightened, the department played a budgetary and managerial shell game, moving key personnel from one grant to another in order to preserve in-house expertise. Federal grants accounted for more than 25% of the department's expenditures for central management during the 1990s.

By quietly siphoning time and resources for essential planning and evaluation activities from federally funded programs, senior managers hoped to maintain the administrative capacity of their programs. The department's success in competing for federal grants in trauma system planning, injury prevention, and minority health, however, provided an unstable revenue stream for its regulatory and planning functions, for most grants were narrowly targeted to a particular problem or issue. Furthermore, most federal planning grants were designed to provide "seed money" to expand state administrative capacities; in the long run, the state was expected to assume primary responsibility for funding the new initiatives. Since the state refused to maintain funding for most new programs in the absence of federal funding, however, most capacity-building efforts were short-lived.

A Weak Mandate

The limited autonomy of state officials in regulating health care financing in Rhode Island rests on the weakness of their statutory mandate. Without a strong mandate and legislative support, public officials in negotiated regimes find it difficult to force private interests to accept changes that do not enjoy universal support from their members. Even where public officials have possessed a strong statutory mandate to regulate the behavior of health care providers, the hospital industry has vigorously opposed efforts to expand the state's regulatory powers. Furthermore, as Rhode Island's experience with the CONCAP demonstrated, unless public officials are firmly committed to cost containment as a primary policy objective, regulatory powers can easily be revoked by legislators in response to pressure from societal interests. While public officials in Rhode Island favor policies to control health care costs, few sought to challenge the professional autonomy of health care providers in order to accomplish this over the past twenty-five years.

The political fortunes of the Maxicap and the CONCAP are closely tied to the scope of their legislative mandate over health care providers. From its inception, the CON process in Rhode Island has been managed by professional careerists within the Department of Health, who operated under a clear grant of statutory authority to regulate facilities construction and service expansion. Over time, the department's pursuit of cost containment through the denial or modification of hospital expansion plans created a plethora of political enemies and few friends.

In contrast, the Maxicap relies on an informal patchwork of public and private interests to negotiate a mutually agreeable forecast of hospital expenditures for the coming year. While the state is represented at all negotiations, much of the burden of budgetary analysis, as well as the substantive issues associated with negotiating individual hospital budgets, falls upon Blue Cross personnel. While conflict is not absent from the process, most conflicts occur between Blue Cross and HARI representatives. Furthermore, unlike the CONCAP process, in which state officials regularly opposed projects that were popular with local communities and their legislative representatives, the Maxicap negotiations are highly technical and largely shrouded from public view.

In the case of the Maxicap, the ambiguity of the enabling legislation has been a political asset, for it did not commit the state to a particular reimbursement methodology. Although no hospital has ever tested the legality of the budget process, the exact requirements imposed on the hospital industry remain unclear twenty years after the state first embraced prospective payment. The essential elements of Rhode Island's prospective payment system are contained in two amendments to the original 1939 act governing Blue Cross. As HARI's legal counsel noted in a 1986 memorandum,

> These two sections set forth an incredibly sparse statutory framework for determining hospital reimbursement. The sections were drafted before the Maxicap was invented and do not mention that concept at all. The statute contemplated individual hospital negotiations. The law purported to require "budget negotiations" held for the purpose of determining payment rates for hospital costs but was (and still is) silent as to the nature of the budgets to be negotiated and as to the methodology by which such budgets are to yield rates. That is, the statute does not require the submission of allowable costs through the Medicare-type cost-finding process, handling of free care, volume corridors, or any of the other baggage which goes along with the process as it has developed (HARI 1986).

In addition, the relationship between the system's principal cost-control agents, the state's budget officer (or his representative), and Blue Cross remains ambiguous. The enabling legislation's only instructions are that representatives from both Blue Cross and the state

> shall be parties to budget negotiations held for the purpose of determining payment rates for hospital costs by the state and such [hospital service]corporations. . . . [S]uch negotiations shall begin no later than ninety days prior to the beginning of each hospital fiscal year. The parties may employ mediation and conciliation services as an aid to such negotiations (R. I. General Laws, § 27-19-14).

Without a clear mandate from the legislature to challenge the autonomy of the hospital industry, the state depends upon Blue Cross representatives to enforce fiscal discipline upon individual hospitals. In effect, the day-to-day management of the state's prospective reimbursement system has been delegated to private groups operating under a grant of public authority. In addition, since state officials are in effect "junior partners" in the Maxicap negotiations, the state cannot adopt a confrontational stance toward HARI or its members without the backing of Blue Cross.

Since its beginning, Rhode Island's certificate-of-need process had a stronger statutory mandate than its rate-setting methodology. Early forays into health care planning bore a strong resemblance to the corporatist system of interest intermediation which produced the Maxicap in the early 1970s. The legislature's decision to regulate capital costs in 1968 followed the recommendations of the Brosco Commission's final report and won endorsements from hospitals and third-party insurers. At the time, hospitals viewed CON as a less onerous alternative to rate-setting, despite the inherent risks of ceding regulatory powers to the state. Furthermore, hospitals, health insurers, and other community groups had previously collaborated in local and regional facilities planning under the aegis of the state's Health Planning Council, a quasi-public body including representatives from all of the core constituencies in the state's health care policy-issue network. In contrast to the state's experience with rate-setting, however, Rhode Island's regulation of hospital capital expenditures evolved from a quasi-public planning process dominated by Blue Cross and the hospital industry to a highly institutionalized system administered by the Department of Health.

TENSIONS WITHIN RHODE ISLAND'S HEALTH CARE-POLICY REGIME

The recurring tensions within the state's policy regime are particularly evident in (1) the administration of the Maxicap, (2) the fate of the Department of Health's draft state health plan in the early 1980s, and (3) the demise of the CONCAP in the early 1990s. Although none of the principal stakeholders in Rhode Island's health care policy regime has pressed for fundamental overhaul of the principles and norms that govern policy-making, tensions have not been absent from either the rate-setting or certificate-of-need programs. In particular, state efforts to rationalize the delivery of health care services by eliminating "excess capacity" aroused intense opposition from health care providers during the 1980s. The CONCAP, in turn, was strongly criticized by HARI and its members as an intrusive policy instrument which imposed significant financial and administrative hardships upon hospitals seeking to upgrade their aging physical plants. Disagreements over the Maxicap have been infrequent. However, HARI and its member hospitals have refused to accept the existing framework of a negotiated global budget as legally binding. Instead, HARI officials contend that while hospitals have voluntarily participated in the Maxicap process to promote efficiency in the health care system, neither the administration of the Maxicap process nor the reimbursement methodology used in the negotiations are specified by the enabling legislation.

The ambiguity regarding the administration of the prospective payment program has often led to tension between Blue Cross and state officials. In the Maxicap's early years, several institutions required the services of a mediator before reaching agreement with Blue Cross, and several hospitals entered the arbitration phase in the 1970s.[14] Indeed, officials within DHS contend that fiscal pressures and increasing competition among Rhode Island's health insurers changed Blue Cross' orientation during the late 1980s. As the former chief of the Department of Human Services' Medicaid bureau noted, "There's a political difference between Blue Cross and the state, and even though we're a team according to the statute, it doesn't always play out that way." The introduction of competition in the state's health insurance market during the early 1980s placed Blue Cross in a precarious fiscal position by the end of the decade. At the same time, Blue Cross had to cope with threats from several hospitals to terminate their contracts in 1990 unless the company approved higher budgets in individual hospital negotiations. While such threats could be disastrous for the defecting hospitals, whose patients would have to seek reimbursement from Blue Cross themselves, they carried weight with Blue Cross officials who were anxious to preserve the company's deteriorating market share. In response, the company adopted an increasingly accommodative stance toward hospitals in order to shore up its sagging enrollments.

The state, for its part, has no fear that it will lose Medicaid beneficiaries to competing insurers and, as a result, is less sensitive to the importance of maintaining smooth relationships with providers. Without full-time staff assigned to manage the Maxicap process, the Department of Human Services has a limited ability to manage the content of the annual budget negotiations or to develop alternative policy options for controlling costs (e.g., a DRG system). Overall, however, disputes among the parties in the Maxicap process are the exception, not the rule. The system virtually runs itself, for as one senior executive for a large urban hospital noted, "We've all been through this drill before."

In contrast, Rhode Island's health planning and CON processes have frequently drawn the ire of providers over the past two decades. Although many groups have supported health facilities planning in Rhode Island over the past thirty years, private or quasi-public planning efforts have been preferred to state-led initiatives. Private planning programs, however, have been plagued by recurring tensions between payers and providers. These cleavages were evident during the state's first excursion into health planning, when the Health Planning Council (HPC), the forerunner of the current Health Services Council, aroused the ire of providers in the late 1960s. From its inception, the council provided a forum for local and regional planning efforts as a quasi-public body of providers, third-party payers, and representatives from various state agencies. The Health Planning Council, however, self-destructed after repeated conflicts between Blue Cross and the state's hospitals over its proper role. Blue Cross kept "banging the hospitals over the head [with cost-containment proposals] and they paid for it," recalled a senior Department of Health official. In the end, hospitals, tired of footing the bill for activities that did not serve their interests, withdrew their support.

The department's political naiveté was reflected in the development of the state's first comprehensive health plan, which proposed a radical restructuring of health care delivery in Rhode Island. The plan proposed, for example, to eliminate "excess capacity" in the state's hospital bed supply and to restrict the number of surgeons who could practice in the state. The draft health plan was released to the public in 1980 and immediately agitated providers, who drummed up support in their local communities to meet the perceived threat (Rochefort and Pezza 1992). The public forums over the draft health plan were raucous affairs that drew hundreds of local residents; at one meeting in southern Rhode Island, local police were called to escort the planners out of town after a tumultuous hearing in which angry residents denounced the state's proposal for closing "surplus" hospitals, a move which would result in layoffs for hundreds of local residents. Employees and patients from hospitals targeted for closure or service reductions jammed public hearings across the state to plead their case (Rochefort and Pezza 1992). After a dose of political reality, the department's subsequent plans backed away from some of its more controversial proposals. Rather than decertifying beds, the department allowed market forces to transform the state's hospital industry during the 1980s.

Nowhere was the push for expanded state authority over health care providers more visible than in the state's CON process. Unlike the Maxicap, the CON process is administered by the Department of Health and an appointed citizens advisory board, the state Health

Services Council. The adversarial, rather than collaborative, nature of the CON process in Rhode Island illustrates the shallow support for state-sponsored regulatory solutions to rising health care costs. HARI has consistently opposed cost-control strategies that do not incorporate provider representatives as active participants in the regulatory decision-making process. The CONCAP process—and CON in general—was viewed as a threat by the industry because it enabled state officials to influence the timing and direction of institutional long-term strategic planning. In a shifting health care market, providers correctly perceived the Health Services Council's emphasis on "affordability" and "public need" as a threat to their institutional autonomy. Unlike the Maxicap negotiations, providers seeking certificate-of-need approval for projects subject to CONCAP review had little institutional leverage over the Department of Health or the Health Services Council.

Hospital displeasure with the CONCAP process stemmed from two important internal contradictions in the legislation itself. First, HARI and other critics point out that while the CONCAP sets a limit on aggregate capital expenditures in a given year, a mismatch exists between capital costs incurred in an upcoming year as defined by the CONCAP and the annualized costs of large capital projects, which often have a lagged effect on hospital revenues several years later (HARI 1986, 10). Second, unlike the Maxicap, the CONCAP process was fraught with uncertainty for hospitals. As a former HARI vice-president argued, "When we go into the CONCAP negotiation process, we go in without knowing what's approved and what's unapproved up front [for the next fiscal year]." The CONCAP also contained a loophole that can provide certain hospitals with an advantage in securing approval for capital projects. If a hospital requests an "expeditious review" of its application, its application automatically moves to the top of the list of potential projects. While the expeditious-review provisions were originally designed to cope with emergency contingencies (e.g., equipment failures or natural disasters), hospitals soon discovered that seeking an expeditious review for projects often increased their chances of approval.

The CONCAP survived for several years without major revisions. The active participation of former legislators such as Representative Anthony Carceri (the architect of the CONCAP) on the state Health Services Council provided CON with legitimacy and helped the department to rebut contentions of hospitals that the process was overly burdensome. From 1987 to 1992, the General Assembly made several changes in the CON statute, largely technical in nature which shortened the review process for proposed projects and raised the financial threshold for project review.[15] By the late 1980s, the Department of Health faced an uphill battle to preserve its CON activities, and political support for CON continued to diminish in the early 1990s. The ongoing opposition of the health care industry was amplified by a growing antiregulatory sentiment in the state's business community, whose leaders expressed growing concerns about the "anti-business reputation" of the state.[16]

Although the high profile of capital projects for local hospitals and communities frequently led to grass-roots campaigns and legislative intervention on behalf of projects under review, by the early 1990s both hospitals and the public regarded the HSC as an organization driven by political rather than policy considerations (Freyer 1993). In 1993, legislators appointed nine new members to the HSC. To make matters worse, two long-time members were abruptly replaced amid a heated discussion over a proposal to build a rehabilitation hospital in Warwick. Less than six months later, three members were replaced during an acrimonious debate over a proposed outpatient surgical center which St. Joseph's Hospital strongly opposed. To further complicate matters, the HSC began issuing decisions based on what appeared to be incompatible objectives. In approving a proposed surgical center in Providence, the HSC dismissed the concerns of hospitals about the "cream-skimming" of patients by citing the virtues of consumer choice and competition. Less than a year later, however, the HSC rejected a similar surgical center in the town of Johnston, citing concerns about the effects of competition on St. Joseph Hospital. Outraged hospital administrators claimed that the process, which in their eyes had always been flawed, now lacked even the semblance of legitimacy.

In 1994, Governor Bruce Sundlun asked the director of health to prepare legislation to modify the CON process. The Sundlun administration was increasingly concerned about the state's slow rate of economic growth. In this climate, the governor viewed CON as a burden for one of the few growth industries in the state (Hackey and Fuller 1995). After a series of meetings between the Department of Health staff and the governor's office, the Sundlun administration drafted legislation that significantly revised the CON process by eliminating the CONCAP. The bill (94-S-2830) was introduced as part of the governor's legislative package and passed the General Assembly with little opposition near the end of the 1994 legislative session. Although the type of projects subject for review by the Health Services Council remain essentially unchanged, the number of projects eligible for approval under the revised statute is unlimited. The General Assembly's action, at the governor's request, had "pulled the teeth of the CON program" in the words of a former Department of Health official.

The demise of the CONCAP illustrates the limits of policy-making under a negotiated regime, for in the absence of support from private peak associations, public initiatives to control health care costs are vulnerable. Furthermore, programs which lack legitimacy in the eyes of key stakeholders in the health care policy-issue network are unlikely to win approval or, if enacted, will become targets for both legal and legislative challenges to circumscribe their authority over affected interests. The growing hostility of hospitals toward a process that most administrators viewed as irrational, inflexible, and arbitrary overcame the limited enthusiasm of state officials to control health care costs through facilities regulation. While negotiated regimes may occasionally challenge the prerogatives of private stakeholders, state officials will find it difficult to sustain such efforts in the long run in the face of significant opposition from private interests.

On several occasions, the cohesion of the state's hospital industry has been splintered by internal divisions over the allocation of funds or the approval of new capital projects. Competition among hospitals for market share intensified considerably during the 1980s, culminating in the merger of two of the state's weaker hospitals (Notre Dame in Central Falls and Fogarty in North Smithfield) with larger institutions in neighboring communities. By 1989, Rhode Island's hospital industry was losing money at a record pace and there were real concerns that one or more of the state's largest urban teaching hospitals might close its doors.[17] In New Jersey, a similar crisis led to a restructuring of its hospital financing system during both the 1970s and 1990s, but Rhode Island legislators responded to the industry's pleas for help with a one-time infusion of cash to particularly hard-hit institutions (Wielawski, Sullivan, and Gregg 1989).

The bailout was initially proposed by St. Joseph's Hospital, a large inner-city teaching hospital which served some of Providence's poorest neighborhoods. Under pressure from the Diocese of Providence, state officials tentatively agreed to allow St. Joseph's to tap into a state fund for hospital construction projects to stem its mounting deficit. When word of the proposed bailout reached the state's other hospitals, hospital administrators and the press were outraged; each institution demanded a piece of the action. As one HARI executive recalled, the bailout "was not our idea. My advice to the hospitals was to walk away from it, but [they] were hurting. The end result was that [the state] gave us $3.5 million of our own money which theoretically should have been plowed back into hospital projects." Initially, the administration of Governor Edward DiPrete proposed to use funds from a quasi-public state agency to offset losses from free care and bad debt at nine nonprofit hospitals. After howls of objection from hospitals excluded from the initial funding formula, however, the proposal evolved into a classic case of distributive politics. Under the new formula proposed by the governor's office, all hospitals qualified for a one-time state grant that was linked to the amount of uncompensated care each institution provided to patients in the previous fiscal year. The state's commitment to alleviating the uncompensated care burden for Rhode Island hospitals, however, was short-lived; unlike Massachusetts, New Jersey, and New York, the Rhode Island legislature made no effort to establish an uncompensated care trust fund to defray the cost of indigent care. Furthermore, although HARI and its members supported a tax on hospital revenues as a means to maximize federal Medicaid reimbursement, no new state strategy to aid distressed hospitals had emerged by the middle of the decade.

The most recent controversy in Rhode Island, however, involved the proposed sale of Roger Williams Medical Center (RWMC) to Columbia/HCA for $51.1 million in 1996. The state's largest newspaper condemned the sale, citing concerns about Columbia/HCA's "checkered history of serving the public" and fears among "many in the Rhode Island health care community . . . that the entry of a for-profit hospital would dismantle what had been a highly efficient and community-oriented hospital system" (*Providence Journal-Bulletin* 1996). The debate over the RWMC deal soon resembled a "who's who" of elected officials, pundits, and public interest groups in the state. Both of the state's Democratic members of the U.S. House of Representatives joined unions, former legislators, social workers, and hospital executives in opposing "Wall Street" health care and "corporate raiders . . . storm[ing] the boardrooms of our struggling health care facilities" (Selya 1996; Coyne-McKay 1996). The early months of 1997 featured a flurry of op-ed pieces decrying the sale, followed by a series of rebuttals from supporters and advocates of competition. In an effort to thwart the move, legislators also rushed to draft legislation that would impose a moratorium on hospital ownership changes, bar the sale of nonprofit hospitals to for-profit chains, and establish a study commission to assess the impact of for-profit hospitals on Rhode Island's health care system (McKay 1997). The introduction of for-profit hospitals also brought new players into health care policy-making circles and thrust decision-making, which had largely been conducted in private negotiations among payers, providers, and state officials or in low-visibility administrative forums (e.g., CON application hearings), onto the front pages of local newspapers. In January and February of 1997 Attorney General Jeffrey Pine held a series of public hearings to gather testimony on the sale, while informational meetings open to the community drew crowds of more than 250 people, most of whom vocally opposed the sale. In the end, the specter of Columbia/HCA's entry into the Rhode Island health care market is likely increased dissension within the membership of the Hospital Association of Rhode Island and raised calls for increased state regulation of the hospital industry. As the chair of the Senate's Corporations Committee observed, "If for-profit medicine is going to come to the state in a big way, then there are definitely going to have to be some new laws" (quoted in McKay 1997, A8).

CONCLUSION

Rhode Island's experience with capital expenditure regulation, rate-setting, and health planning over the past three decades illustrates both the perils and possibilities of policy-making under a negotiated regime. While hospitals have frequently expressed displeasure with certain aspects of the state's cost-containment strategy, neither providers nor payers have mounted a judicial challenge to the legitimacy of the state's rate-setting or certificate-of-need programs. Both HARI and Blue Cross and Blue Shield of Rhode Island continue to support the Maxicap process as a decentralized and effective means of controlling costs. The delegation of significant administrative authority to key stakeholders also permitted the process to respond to changing market conditions over time and to accommodate the unique needs of individual institutions within an overall expenditure target.

Rhode Island's experience with CON and rate-setting over the past two decades illustrates the limits of regulation in states that lack the institutional capacity to administer and update complex regulatory programs. Weak political institutions handicapped the efforts of state officials to develop more comprehensive reforms of the hospital payment system. State officials from the Department of Human Services served as junior partners in a private negotiating process between Blue Cross and the Hospital Association of Rhode Island and lacked the ability to gather essential information, analyze the fiscal impacts of new expenditures, or develop alternatives to the current system. In the end, public officials lacked the tools to discipline the hospital industry and depended on voluntary cooperation from HARI and the expertise and bargaining power of Blue Cross to control costs. Hospitals opposed the state's reformed certificate-of-need process on the grounds that it was biased and unnecessarily restricted the ability of hospital administrators to react to changes in health care organization and delivery. Nevertheless, HARI and its members have not pressed for a repeal of all state authority to review capital projects; hospital displeasure with the CONCAP stemmed from its perceived shortcomings and did not reflect an overall hostility toward any state intervention in health care financing.

The public-private partnership at the core of Rhode Island's rate-setting process offers an instructive lesson for other states. Two decades of experience with the Maxicap demonstrate that expenditure limitations for health care services need not require an extensive administrative apparatus in order to control costs. Furthermore, the active incorporation of private stakeholders in both the formulation and implementation of the Maxicap provided the state's cost-containment efforts with a strong base of political support and added legitimacy to the decision-making process in the eyes of providers and third-party payers. Without support from private groups, negotiated regimes are ill-equipped to sustain cost-containment policies, for disaffected stakeholders are often able to thwart policies which challenge the autonomy or prerogatives of providers or payers.

The stability of Rhode Island's negotiated health care policy regime can also be traced to an absence of external pressures for reform. Health care policy-making in Rhode Island continues to be dominated by the same groups that created the state's prospective payment system in the early 1970s. Unlike other states, no new groups have emerged as significant actors in the state's health care policy-issue network, which remains impermeable to potentially destabilizing influences representing consumers, labor, or the business community. As a result, policy-making on most issues is shaped by two competing advocacy coalitions: on the one hand, hospitals press for additional resources and seek to limit outside competition, while Blue Cross supports efforts by the Health Department and the Department of Human Services to control costs. To date, neither the state's hospitals nor Blue Cross have faced a sustained fiscal crisis that might open the door to the expansion of state authority over heath care financing. In the absence of fundamental changes in the fiscal health of Rhode Island's hospitals, the state is unlikely to press for a new system of financing or regulatory controls.

Health care policy-making in Rhode Island has remained nonideological and nonpartisan over the past two decades. Candidates for the governorship, in particular, have conducted pragmatic campaigns that emphasized ethics and economic growth; the election of Republican governors in 1984 and 1994 had few consequences for the state's health care policy regime, as neither Edward DiPrete nor Lincoln Almond relied heavily upon ideological appeals. Solid Democratic control over the General Assembly eliminated another agent of policy transformation; in the absence of serious opposition, the Democratic leadership had few incentives to uproot long-standing policy-making arrangements such as the Maxicap. In addition, since the legality of Rhode Island's regulatory apparatus has not been tested in court, judges have had no opportunities to remake the state's health care financing system.

The likelihood of significant changes in the relationship between state officials and private groups within Rhode Island's health care policy regime appears low for the foreseeable future. Despite the state's recent embrace of managed care as a means of controlling Medicaid costs, public officials, health care providers, and third-party payers continue to support the state's collaborative approach to cost-containment. Until the proposed acquisition of Roger Williams' Medical Center in 1996, health care policy-making remained a low-profile issue in Rhode Island for lawmakers. Legislators' attention in recent years has been focused upon economic development, ethical reforms, the deregulation of electric utilities, and options for addressing the state's chronic structural budget deficit. The unusual public-private partnership governing hospital reimbursement and health care planning in Rhode Island reflects the intimacy of the state's tightly knit policy network. Since the expectations, norms, and actors involved in shaping the health care policy agenda have changed little over the past two decades, few external pressures for change exist in Rhode Island. Furthermore, aside from the state's ten-year experiment with the CONCAP, few internal contradictions threaten the interests of key actors, for the consultative nature of policy-making in Rhode Island ensures that most disputes are resolved through corporatist bargaining or by incorporating affected interests in the implementation of the state's cost-containment efforts. The end result of the state's meso-corporatist approach to cost control, however, is a unique system which enjoys strong support from its principal stakeholders.

CHAPTER NOTES

1. As HARI officials are quick to point out, however, the precise obligations of hospitals under the "sparse" statutory framework governing prospective reimbursement in Rhode Island remain unclear. Although the requirement to negotiate annual budgets has never been challenged in court, since the enabling legislation was drafted prior to the development of the Maxicap process, it is not clear whether or not hospitals are legally bound to the existing framework (Hospital Association of Rhode Island 1986).

2. The Women and Infants' project became politicized early in the CON process, since its focus on maternal health and the determination of pregnancy made it the largest provider of obstetrical services (and hence abortions) in the most Catholic state in the nation. The proposed project pointed out a glaring weakness of the state's cost-control process—there was a disjunction between the state's health planning and cost-control objectives. Since additional facilities and services raise the cost of hospital care, state officials decided to pursue an aggressive strategy to limit new construction.

3. The Health Care System Affordability Act increased the threshold for CON review from $150,000 for capital projects and $75,000 for increases in operating costs. In practice, however, the legislation covered nearly all capital projects, for even the replacement of a hospital's telephone or management information systems regularly exceeded the review threshold.

4. Under the terms of the 1984 legislation, total expenditures for capital projects (including interest and depreciation) in any fiscal year may not exceed four tenths of one percent (0.04) of the total operating expenditures for all hospitals in the state.

5. Negotiations center around what are reasonable estimates for inflation in each category of the Maxicap, based on both estimates of overall expected inflation drawn from econometric models provided by the state's DRI/Mc-Graw-Hill forecasts and projected increases in FICA, unemployment insurance, worker's compensation, health insurance, and other costs.

6. Indeed, the process recognizes that circumstances beyond a hospital's control may cause it to exceed its negotiated budget. To provide for unforeseen expenses, each Maxicap includes a prespecified reserve in its global expense budget. In past years, unanticipated increases in malpractice insurance premiums for hospitals were regarded as major contingencies under which hospitals could legitimately seek adjustments to their negotiated budgets.

7. According to HARI officials, this approach was copied from Charlie Finley's negotiations of baseball contracts for the Oakland A's in the 1970s.

8. Volume corridors had their origins in the managerial and staffing problems facing hospitals, for costs associated with increased patient volume often exceed increases in marginal costs. In most cases, hospitals are able to absorb minor changes in volume without adding additional personnel or opening new floors. However, as one hospital executive noted, "You either add or don't add [personnel] to open a unit, floor, or wing. Minimum staffing requirements must be met."

9. The capital-expense ratio describes the cost of interest and depreciation relative to an institution's total operating expenses; since higher values for the ratio indicate a higher level of indebtedness, lower values are indicative of both fiscal health and fewer long-term obligations.

10. Donald Brand (1988, 20) defines administrative corporatism as "an institutionalized pattern of administration in which groups monopolistically represent interests and where they play a significant role (formal or informal) in policymaking and policy implementation."

11. For a more complete discussion of the Nixon administration's economic stabilization plan, see Kosters (1975).

12. Only self-paying patients and the Workers' Compensation fund were excluded.

13. As Cornwell and Moakley (1996) note, in recent years the ability of bill sponsors to have their bills heard in committee has increased as a result of recent rules changes. Furthermore, the 1990s reforms also permitted members to attempt to override unfavorable committee actions on the floor and extended the time between committee consideration and floor votes to permit more discussion of the merits of various policy proposals.

14. The CONCAP section of the Maxicap negotiations has been submitted to binding arbitration twice since 1984. In the most recent case, the arbitrator sided with HARI's contention that the CONCAP proposed by Blue Cross and the state ($4 million) in 1992 was inadequate to fund the number of projects proposed; the arbitrator agreed to HARI's request for a $5.5 million CONCAP for the 1992 review cycle.

15. The amendments during this period raised the state's CON review thresholds to reflect changes in federal standards and exempted health maintenance organizations from CON review prior to licensing (Pub. L. 1985, Chapter 500). Subsequent changes allowed for a three-year transition period to the new CON thresholds (Pub. L. 1986, Chapter 363) and shortened the maximum length of the review process for projects subject to CONCAP limitations (Pub. L. 1987, Chapter 395).

16. In a series of reports, the Rhode Island Public Expenditure Council, a well-respected business-sponsored watchdog group, repeatedly cited excessive government regulation as a disincentive for business to move to the state and a liability for the state's efforts to retain existing firms and encourage job creation.

17. The state's fourteen private hospitals posted a loss of more than $30 million in FY1988. This situation improved somewhat in 1989, when eight hospitals reported losses of more than $22 million. By 1990, the fiscal health of the state's hospital industry was considerably stronger, as the combined losses among the state's private hospitals had fallen to $5.1 million (Wielawski, Sullivan, and Gregg 1989).

6

New Hampshire: Private Solutions for Public Problems

New Hampshire has pursued a market-oriented strategy in health care for more than three decades. Aside from the state's CON process, public officials possess little or no formal authority to regulate the hospital industry. Hospitals are free to negotiate contracts with health insurers as they see fit, although insurers' premiums are subject to review by the state's insurance commissioner. In addition, an ideological consensus among both public and private participants in the political process strongly supports privately administered solutions to control health care costs. The delegation of reimbursement decisions to the private sector, in turn, minimizes conflict between state officials and the hospital industry, for most decisions emerge as a by-product of contract negotiations between health care providers and third-party payers.

The state's preference for market-based initiatives to control health care costs is also reflected in efforts by state officials to promote competition among health care providers and health insurers. In 1996, New Hampshire applied for a statewide managed care waiver to enroll all AFDC-eligible Medicaid beneficiaries in managed care plans as a means of controlling program costs without resorting to extensive government price setting. Fostering competition among health care providers for paying patients has also been the principal goal of the state's certificate-of-need process over the past decade. Neither state officials nor private groups, however, have seriously considered more active government involvement to increase access to health care or control costs through rate-setting, global budgeting, or the creation of state-funded uncompensated care pools. Instead, the state's policy options are defined by New Hampshire's intensely conservative political culture: an expanded state role in health care financing, or other areas of social policy, lacks legitimacy in the eyes of the public and commands no support among elected officials and key interest groups.

Prospects for significant changes in New Hampshire's market-based regime appear dim for the foreseeable future, as both public and private elites express confidence in the state's "hands off" approach to controlling health care costs. Tensions within the regime remain limited in duration and scope, as contract disputes among providers and third-party payers, or between providers seeking to offer similar services, have not polarized key interests into competing advocacy coalitions. Although it remains overbedded, New Hampshire's hospital industry has not experienced a wrenching fiscal crisis in response to the steady increase in the number of residents enrolled in managed care plans. Furthermore, since the state has never regulated hospital rates or imposed significant restrictions on the managerial autonomy of health care providers, neither hospitals nor insurers are pressing for a change in state policy. In the absence of state initiatives to remake the health care financing system, providers and businesses have collaborated on several ventures to coordinate the delivery of high-cost services and expand access to vulnerable populations and rural communities. In lieu of state-funded initiatives to increase access to health care, public officials in New Hampshire have recently expressed interest in establishing a "volunteer clearinghouse" to coordinate the delivery of *pro bono* services to the medically indigent.

THE POLICY-MAKING ENVIRONMENT IN NEW HAMPSHIRE

New Hampshire's population of 1.1 million is served by 26 community hospitals; Dartmouth-Hitchcock Medical Center, the state's largest teaching hospital, is one of the state's five largest employers. The industry, however, remains significantly overbedded. Although the state's ratio of hospital beds per 1,000 residents was the lowest in New England, the average occupancy rate barely exceeded 50% in 1992. The low level of utilization reflects the state's rural character, for fifteen of the state's acute-care hospitals have fewer than one hundred beds and many are located in remote areas in the northern and western areas of the state. The hospital industry in New Hampshire is in strong fiscal health despite an acknowledged surplus of beds. The industry's fiscal position improved dramatically in the early 1990s as a result of a $47 million windfall obtained as a result of the state's efforts to maximize federal reimbursement for institutions that treated a "disproportionate share" of Medicaid patients in 1991 (Jimenez 1992a). Despite a regional recession, New Hampshire hospitals' revenues exceeded expenditures by $72 million in 1992; the industry's median operating margin in 1992 (0.054) was one of the highest operating margins in the nation (Boston Globe 1992; Cleverly 1993).

Unlike other states, the New Hampshire Hospital Association's (NHHA) role has receded in recent years, as decisions by the state's insurance commissioner strengthened the hand of Blue Cross officials at the expense of the state's hospital industry. Hospitals have had a close working relationship with physicians and the business community; collaborative approaches to decision-making and coordination of services are commonplace. Unlike New York and Massachusetts, where businesses became active participants in the legislative process in an effort to control rising health care costs, business groups in New Hampshire have participated in joint planning efforts aimed at improving the efficiency of the health care system without public intervention. In recent years, hospitals have embraced collaborative planning and service coordination to offer mobile MRI and lithotripsy services. As Ron Sliwinksi, a vice president at Mary Hitchcock Memorial Hospital noted, "It makes all the sense in the world to coordinate services and cooperate in high-technology ventures and not to duplicate ourselves so much that we're fighting for the same patients" (quoted in Cerne 1993, 50). Increasing vertical and horizontal integration of health care facilities has also occurred in New Hampshire in the 1990s. Several hospitals have merged in recent years and one of the state's largest hospitals (Mary Hitchcock Memorial) was acquired by an HMO, Matthew Thornton Health Plan. In 1994, Manchester's Elliot Hospital formed a new partnership, Optima Health, with Catholic Medical Center in Manchester; the new network soon formed affiliations with several community hospitals in Portsmouth, Exeter, and Derry (Jimenez 1994b).

Hospital reimbursement in the Granite State remains a private process, largely free from government intervention or direct regulation. The state's insurance commissioner has a limited role in the reimbursement process by reviewing proposed rate increases for Blue Cross subscribers, but reimbursement for acute-care hospital services is determined by individual negotiations between hospitals and third-party payers. No parameters or guidelines for reimbursement negotiations are established by the state, nor do providers have access to state funds to offset the costs of free care and bad debt. Both the hospitals and the payers express satisfaction with the present system; neither group expressed support for a larger government role. Since neither payers nor hospitals have found themselves in extreme financial difficulty in recent years, few external pressures exist to reconfigure the present privately controlled system.

New Hampshire's principal third-party payers include Blue Cross, Medicaid, Medicare, two HMOs, and several commercial insurers. The insurance market is highly competitive; while none of the commercial insurers has a large share of the market, several companies have established a foothold in the state. Blue Cross, however, is by far the most significant payer in the system; with 23% of the state's population enrolled as subscribers, it controls almost one-half of the nongovernment health insurance market. Blue Cross occupies center stage in debates over hospital reimbursement issues. Significantly, more than 50% of the state's businesses remain self-insured (Cerne 1993). In the absence of a significant state presence, and with little legislative activity on the part of businesses, physicians, or other groups, health care financing issues continue to be dominated by Blue Cross. In 1996, Blue Cross and Blue Shield of New Hampshire announced plans to join a regional alliance sponsored by Blue Cross and Blue Shield of Massachusetts to jointly market their products to customers in the region.

Enrollment in managed care organizations has more than doubled since 1989; 22% of the state's population (240,000 people) were covered by a managed care plan in 1995, an increase of nearly 25% from 1994 (Globe 1996a). By the end of 1996, more than 300,000 New Hampshire residents were enrolled in the state's two largest HMOs—Healthsource, a for-profit HMO, had more than 170,000 members, while Matthew Thornton Health Plan enrolled an additional 139,000 residents (Pham 1996a). New Hampshire, however, had the highest percentage of uninsured residents under age 65 of any state in New England from 1990 to 1992 (Kaiser Commission 1995a). Health care costs are low relative to both regional and national averages, for New Hampshire residents are the healthiest in the nation; per capita spending on hospital care is far below the New England average, as is hospital utilization (Jimenez 1995). HMOs negotiate their own contracts with providers, typically as a discount off of the hospital's charges, but their relationship with the hospital industry does not extend beyond their individual contracts with providers. Further changes in the state's health care marketplace loom on the horizon, as Matthew Thornton Health Plan entered into negotiations to merge with Harvard Pilgrim Health Care in 1996 after a previous merger attempt failed in 1994.

Apart from their role as purchasers of care, business organizations have assumed a low profile in health care policy-making in New Hampshire. Corporate executives have followed a private approach to managing rising health care costs rather than seeking public solutions. Since hospital reimbursement remains a private process, few opportunities exist for public review and commentary on health care financing matters. As a result, businesses have few incentives to lobby the legislature on health policy matters, for lawmakers have considered few significant health care reform proposals in recent years. Despite rising costs, business leaders have not adopted a confrontational stance toward the hospital industry. As the president of the Business and Industry Association of New Hampshire noted, businesses are "not going to talk our way out of a problem that we behaved our way into. The fact is that everyone in the equation has to change their behavior; we need to change the way we purchase health care and change the way it is delivered" (quoted in Cerne 1993, 51). Businesses have expressed considerable interest in benefits management and "prudent purchasing" arrangements to control costs, but have not enlisted support from state legislators or the governor's office to apply public pressure to control hospital expenditures. Demands for change are also notably absent from other interests in New Hampshire; neither labor nor public interest reform groups have emerged as significant players in the policy-making process.

NEW HAMPSHIRE'S APPROACH TO COST CONTAINMENT

New Hampshire's response to inflation in the health sector reflects a shared set of preferences among public officials, private interests, and the public for limited government. For the past three decades, promises to keep state government small, lean, and "off of people's backs" have been a recurrent theme in state elections. With few initiatives forthcoming from the governor's office or the legislature to reform health care financing, decision-making on most issues rests squarely with the private sector. Hospital rates are negotiated through a private bargaining process between health insurers and providers without interference from state officials. While changes in insurer service offerings are subject to approval by the state's Department of Insurance, the department does not participate in negotiations with or approve contracts between the hospitals and third-party payers. Under these circumstances, hospital reimbursement decision-making in New Hampshire resembles Paul Starr's (1982) description of American health policy for much of the twentieth century: public power and authority are ceded to health care providers.

In the words of one senior official at Blue Cross and Blue Shield of New Hampshire, "The only real regulation that's imposed upon the hospitals is the certificate-of-need (CON) process, and that's as criticized here as in any other state where it exists." More than a decade ago, Drew Altman and his co-authors characterized New Hampshire as "a state where planners have yet to develop a clear regulatory strategy" (Altman, Greene, and Sapolsky 1981, 58). Review of hospital capital expenditures began in 1973 under the voluntary process established by Section 1122 of the 1972 Social Security Amendments, but the state was slow to adopt more stringent certificate-of-need controls. Certificate-of-need was not introduced in New Hampshire until 1979, five years after the passage of Pub. L. 93-641. New Hampshire was one of the last states in the nation to implement a certificate-of-need program as required by Pub. L. 93-641. Its conservative Republican governor, Meldrim Thomson, was adamantly opposed to new federal mandates in any form, and the state's attitude toward federally mandated health planning was openly hostile. The state's sole Health Systems Agency lacked support from the governor's office during the administration of Thomson from 1974 to 1978 and did not fully exercise its regulatory powers (Altman, Greene, and Sapolsky 1981, 16).

Data analysis, health planning, and certificate-of-need activities reside within the eleven-member state Health Services Planning and Review Board (HSPRB), which is charged with setting standards "relative to the size, type, level, quality, and affordability of health care services offered in New Hampshire" (New Hampshire Health Services Planning and Review Board 1992, i).[1] Projects subject to CON review in the early 1990s included all new capital construction in excess of $1.5 million, new equipment purchases of $400,000 or more, and any new services that would add to an institution's operating costs.[2]

The authorizing legislation for health planning in the Granite State was passed in 1979, five years after the passage of the National Health Planning and Resources Development Act. Certificate-of-need had an inauspicious beginning in New Hampshire, however, for state officials neglected to define standards of need for new services. The first significant legal challenge to the state's CON statute occurred in 1981, when developers of a new psychiatric hospital challenged the state Office of Health Planning and Development's decision to withdraw a CON permit which it had previously approved. The case provides a unique perspective on the state's implementation of Pub. L. 93-641, for program staff failed to follow the basic statutory requirements imposed by the legislature. In *Appeal of Behavioral Science Institute* in 1981, the state supreme court noted that "by failing to promulgate rules and regulations governing the application process for new health care facilities, the State agency contributed in large part to the pervading confusion in the proceedings. . . ."[3] The court's opinion raised fundamental questions about the capacity of state bureaucrats to undertake their new tasks; as the court observed, the OHPD's handling of the matter was "so replete with error that the decision must be overturned."

Events suggest that the state's CON process continued to suffer from an unusually slow learning curve. In its review of a proposal to convert inpatient substance abuse beds to inpatient psychiatric beds,

HSPRB once again failed to follow the three-step process outlined by the legislature for reviewing new institutional health services, which required the HSPRB to (1) develop standards for services, (2) identify need, and (3) attempt to fill the need. More than a decade after the court's decision in *Appeal of Behavioral Science Institute*, the state continued to make CON decisions without reference to the standards identified in the state's health plan. Furthermore, although New Hampshire's CON statute strongly encouraged competition among providers to offer new services by issuing requests for applications in identified areas of need, the HSPRB failed to issue such a notice. In short, the court's decision suggested that the HSPRB's members and staff were unfamiliar with, or neglected to apply, their own planning guidelines in evaluating competing applications for new services and service conversions (*Appeal of Nashua Brookside Hospital* 1994).

New Hampshire's decision to retain certificate of need after the expiration of federal health planning requirements in 1986 appears to be incongruous with the state's disdain of government regulation. Legislators, however, regarded CON review as a procompetitive policy rather than a coercive regulatory tool. Indeed, the enabling legislation justified the review of institutional health services on the grounds that "the state has an interest in promoting and stimulating competition among providers in the health care marketplace as a means of managing the increases in health care costs" (New Hampshire Revised Statutes Annotated; RSA 151-C:1). The continued presence of CON in New Hampshire, however, reflects providers' view that the review process can be used as a means to defend market share from new competitors. In 1994, legislators recognized that the changing health care marketplace threatened the viability of small community hospitals and several of the state's larger institutions in a little-noticed amendment to the stated goals of the CON process. Rather than encouraging further competition among providers, the amendment declared that the state "has an interest in promoting and stimulating collaboration among providers in the health care marketplace as a means of managing the increase in health care costs" (New Hampshire Revised Statutes Annotated; RSA 151-C:1, III).

The ongoing dispute over cardiac catheterization services between Catholic Medical Center (CMC) and Elliot Hospital in Manchester illustrates how institutions have sought to employ CON as a weapon against potential competitors. Prior to their affiliation in 1994, the two institutions sparred in court for several years over the right of Elliot Hospital to offer left-heart cardiac catheterization services on an outpatient basis. Although the state Supreme Court ultimately rejected CMC's claim that new outpatient services required a CON, both CMC and its fellow plaintiff, Portsmouth Hospital, sought to quash new service offerings by a nearby institution under the aegis of the state's CON statute. In the intensely competitive market for paying patients in New Hampshire, CON is seen as an ally to defend the market share and service areas of local hospitals.

Although the state began paying hospitals prospectively on the basis of diagnosis-related groups (DRGs) in 1989 under the Medicaid program, it did so only after extensive consultation with the New Hampshire Hospital Association. As one of the architects of the new payment system expressed it, "In constructing these final rules [for the PPS/DRG Medicaid system] we attempted to incorporate to the extent possible the recommendations and concerns of our committee/work group. . . . I believe we were largely successful in this effort."[4] Since hospital payment negotiations occur within a private contracting process, without the institutional framework for overseeing and approving the results of the bargaining among private groups, state officials had little opportunity to influence policy.

The state's preferred cost-control strategy over the past decade has been to encourage the growth of market competition among providers by limiting anticompetitive practices and moving Medicaid beneficiaries into managed care. State interventions in private markets, however, do not attempt to "micromanage" the industry. In 1996, legislators justified a prohibition on exclusive contracts between insurers and health care providers on the grounds that "competition is fostered by minimal barriers to entry and exit in the relevant market, and exclusive arrangements between physicians and managed care insurers have effectively created barriers to entry which effectively prevent competing managed care insurers from doing business" (Chapter 134 of the Public Laws of 1996). Furthermore, the legislation emphatically endorsed competition as the state's principal cost-containment tool. In the eyes of the General Court, "Competition among physicians and health care providers, facilities, payers, and purchasers yields the best allocation of health care resources, the lowest prices, and the highest quality of health care."

The cornerstone of New Hampshire's market-oriented approach to health care reform has been the growing importance of Medicaid managed care. Prior to the early 1990s, however, enrollment in Medicaid managed care programs was limited. Beginning in the mid-1980s, the state implemented a clinic-based voluntary managed care program for residents in one geographic area. In 1994, the state expanded opportunities for voluntary enrollment by contracting with a statewide independent practice association. Enrollment for all categories of beneficiaries, however, remained voluntary; the state did not seek a free-dom-of-choice waiver from HCFA to permit mandatory enrollment in MCOs. The state's principal policy initiative in recent years was the development of a statewide Medicaid demonstration waiver applica-tion that was filed in June 1996. Under the terms of its Section 1115 waiver application, New Hampshire proposed to create an integrated delivery system that would provide a continuity of care for poor pa-tients.

The state's proposal, formally known as "Community Care Sys-tems," sought permission to provide capitated managed care services for all AFDC-eligible Medicaid enrollees (State of New Hampshire 1996). In addition, New Hampshire's waiver sought to insulate the state from unanticipated costs as a result of increased program enroll-ment. The state requested that federal participation in the waiver con-tinue up to an aggregate budget limit for five years, with additional federal funds available to the state if actual enrollment exceeds projec-tions by more than 3% per year. Furthermore, the waiver requests permission for the state to retain any "efficiencies and savings in the per capita cost of care" to finance program expansions and/or reduce the state's spending on services. Significantly, however, the state's proposed managed care waiver included no new state funding to in-crease access to care for uninsured or vulnerable populations. Instead, any program expansions will be financed through cost savings gener-ated by a competitive bidding process with MCOs to provide capitated services for the 90,000 eligible program beneficiaries. To date, however, the implementation of managed care as New Hampshire's principal policy lever for controlling Medicaid costs still awaits final approval from HCFA.

The Success of New Hampshire's Cost-Containment Efforts

Facilities planning in New Hampshire has not significantly affected the managerial autonomy of health care providers. The HSPRB's policy of restraint in applying its powers of CON review to reshape the organization and delivery of health care services in New Hampshire is consistent with the state's overall emphasis on markets, rather than regulation, to control health care costs. Since an active CON program restricts the ability of hospitals to respond to changes in physician and patient demand, the state's market regime has frequently accommo-dated the interests of health care providers. In the late 1980s the HSPRB demonstrated its determination to control costs through what one se-nior Blue Cross official described as several "well thought-out denials" that culminated in the rejection of a proposal to construct a new hospital in Portsmouth in 1989. The stringency of the state's review process appeared to increase again in the summer of 1990, when Governor Judd Gregg announced a moratorium on CON petitions; any applications that had been filed at that point were to be considered, but no further applications would be accepted. In the face of lower hospital occupancy rates and rising Medicaid outlays, the HSPRB disallowed more than 50% of the capital expenditures proposed during FY1989 and FY1990.

Without a constraint on overall capital expenditures, however, the HSPRB's performance in controlling capital expenditures over the past decade has been lackluster (see Tables 6.1–6.3). The HSPRB has also failed to slow the diffusion of new technologies through the use of CON review, for without a constraint on overall capital expenditures, few applications were rejected by the HSPRB. In 1982, the board approved seven of the eight applications before it to establish MRI services, and while it denied all four applications to install new MRI facilities in 1985, it subsequently approved six additional units from 1986 to 1991 (see Table 6.2). A similar pattern is evident in the board's actions on the acquisition of CT scanners; the board approved every application for the purchase or lease of CT scanning equipment that was presented from 1976 to 1991. Furthermore, the state's approach to regulating the diffusion of cardiac care services suggests that CON in

TABLE 6.1   Disposition of CON Applications in New Hampshire: Acute-Care Hospital Services

Year	Approved	Withdrawn	Denied	N
1982	7	0	1	8
1983	4	0	2	6
1984	6	0	0	6
1985	4	1	0	5
1986	1	0	0	1
1987	2	2	0	4
1988	6	0	0	6
1989	4	0	2	6
1990	1	0	1	2
1991	4	0	0	4
Total	39	3	6	48
%	81	6	13	100

Source: New Hampshire Department of Health and Human Services

TABLE 6.2   Disposition of CON Applications in New Hampshire: Magnetic Resonance Imaging

Year	Approved	Withdrawn	Denied	N
1982	7	0	1	8
1983	0	0	0	0
1984	0	0	0	0
1985	0	0	4	4
1986	4	0	0	4
1987	1	0	0	1
1988	1	0	0	1
1989	0	0	0	0
1990	0	0	0	0
1991	0	0	0	0
Total	13	0	5	18
%	72	0	28	100

Source: New Hampshire Department of Health and Human Services

New Hampshire was ultimately a procedural "waiting game." Although the HSPRB rejected three of six applications for the development of inpatient cardiac catheterization services in 1988, it subsequently approved each institution's request for reconsideration in the following year.

Aside from the high-profile denials of new construction projects proposed by Elliot Hospital in Manchester and the denial of a CON for a new ninety-bed acute-care hospital in Salem in 1989, the HSPRB has not aggressively challenged the capital spending plans of hospitals. Indeed, while the board rejected all four applications to expand magnetic resonance imaging services it considered in 1985, it subsequently approved each of the four proposals in the following year. Of the 89 hospital-related CON applications reviewed by the HSPRB during the ten-year period from 1982 to 91, 77% (N=69) were approved.

Although CON controls provide only an indirect incentive to control the cost and utilization of health care services, the ineffectiveness of the state's CON review process placed few pressures on hospitals to control costs during the 1980s. From 1983 to 1988, the number of full-time equivalent personnel employed by New Hampshire's hospital industry increased 13.7%, faster than any state in the region and well above the national average; during the same period, the state's ratio of hospital expenses per capita also increased faster than other states

TABLE 6.3   Disposition of CON Applications in New Hampshire: Cardiac Care and CT Scanners

Year	Approved	Withdrawn	Denied	N
1982	0	0	0	0
1983	1	0	0	1
1984	1	1	0	2
1985	5	1	0	6
1986	1	0	0	1
1987	0	0	0	0
1988	3	0	3	6
1989	4	0	0	4
1990	1	1	0	2
1991	1	0	0	1
Total	17	3	3	23
%	74	13	13	100

Source: New Hampshire Department of Health and Human Services

in New England (New Hampshire Hospital Association 1990). Although the overall cost of health care in New Hampshire was low relative to other states in the Northeast (the state ranked 36th in the nation in per capita spending on hospital services in 1994), the rate of inflation was comparable, or higher than, other states in the region during the 1990s (Jensen et. al. 1994, 19). In particular, since New Hampshire lacks any broad-based sales or income taxes to finance state expenditures, Medicaid represented an enormous drain on the state's limited fiscal resources.

In the early 1990s, rising Medicaid costs threatened to shatter the decades-old consensus which had resisted new forms of taxation, for New Hampshire found itself in a Medicaid-induced fiscal crisis during the 1990–92 recession. As the regional economy fell into a tailspin in 1989 and 1990, job losses increased dramatically. The ripple effect of the state's economic malaise was soon felt in both the Medicaid program budget and by community hospitals, which treated an increasing number of medically indigent patients. Medicaid enrollment increased 23.3% in New Hampshire from 1990 to 1992, nearly double the national and regional average for the period. At the same time expenditures (excluding disproportionate-share payments to hospitals) increased by 27.7%, faster than any other state in New England (Winterbottom, Liska, and Obermaier 1995, 127). Rising hospital costs also contributed to a sharp increase in Blue Cross premiums in the late 1980s and early 1990s. After Blue Cross' losses peaked at more than $30 million in 1988, the company petitioned the state insurance commissioner to permit it to abandon its system of "community rated" insurance rates, in which younger and healthier subscribers cross-subsidized the premiums of older and sicker plan members. In an effort to restore Blue Cross to fiscal solvency, the state insurance commissioner granted the company's request to institute a risk-based approach to setting premiums in 1991 that used an individual's age, gender, and job to determine his or her premium rate. As a result, premiums doubled, and in some cases tripled, for "high-risk" subscribers.

A federally financed windfall, however, provided a reprieve for New Hampshire's emerging fiscal crisis. Beginning in the late 1980s, a number of states exploited a loophole that allowed public officials to define which hospitals serve a "disproportionate share" of Medicaid patients; since hospitals that treated a large volume of publicly insured patients frequently had an above-average uncompensated care caseload, Medicaid reimbursement rules allowed designated "disproportionate share hospitals" (DSH) to qualify for additional federal matching payments. Across the U.S., state governments created a wide range of innovative financing arrangements designed to maximize state spending on DSH payments, enabling the states to obtain federal subsidies for expenditures that had previously been state-funded. Although Congress had encouraged states to increase payments to disproportionate-share hospitals as a means of bolstering the health of ailing urban teaching hospitals and other facilities at risk of closure, states quickly recognized that DSH rules offered virtually unlimited opportunities for intergovernmental cost shifting.

No state has exploited the provisions of DSH financing more than New Hampshire; in a single stroke, passage of legislation permitting the state to qualify for enhanced Medicaid reimbursement wiped out a $100 million budget shortfall and provided a transfusion of cash for the state's beleaguered hospitals. Harry Bird, the state's commissioner of Health and Human Services, laid the groundwork for the windfall by classifying all hospitals, nursing homes, and rehabilitation centers in New Hampshire as serving a "disproportionate share" of Medicaid patients. As Commissioner Bird quipped in 1991, "We've got a $100 million problem. Well, I've got a $100 million solution" (quoted in Milne 1991, NH8). The budget-balancing plan offered by Governor Gregg imposed a 30% tax on hospitals' gross receipts, yielding nearly $200 million in new revenues for the state. More than half of the tax revenues were returned to the hospitals in the form of higher state Medicaid reimbursements; hospitals were reimbursed for the remainder through federal matching payments (Milne 1991). Although some cynics in the legislature assailed the Gregg plan as a "gross deceits tax" which blatantly exploited federal Medicaid reimbursement rules to balance the state's budget at Washington's expense, legislators overwhelmingly endorsed the proposal as a means of avoiding new broad-based taxes.

The state's success in squeezing additional federal reimbursement from Medicaid provider taxes is undeniable. By 1993, disproportionate-share payments to providers accounted for more than 50% of all state Medicaid spending, making New Hampshire far and away the national leader in the percentage of Medicaid funds allocated for DSH payments. In addition, New Hampshire's DSH payments per uninsured person were the highest in the United States in 1993 ($2,717) and contributed to an average *annual* growth rate in the state's Medicaid budget of more than 35% from 1988 to 1993 (Kaiser Foundation 1995b, 119). Most of the additional federal funds, however, were not used to extend access to health care for the uninsured, but rather to balance the budgets of the state and participating hospitals (Jimenez 1993). Indeed, excluding disproportionate share payments, state spending on Medicaid actually declined an average of 1.1% per year from 1988 to 1993, making New Hampshire the only state in the nation which spent less per beneficiary in 1993 than it had five years earlier (Kaiser Foundation 1995b, 119). Soon after the money began pouring in, critics accused the state of balancing its budget at the expense of children and the uninsured. Terry Lochhead, the director of the New Hampshire Alliance for Children, assailed the state's DSH program as "a taxing system in which children are trampled in the rush to generate federal funds" (Lochhead 1991). While state officials disagreed with critics' assessment, they did not disavow efforts to swap federal dollars for state funds. As Commissioner Bird observed, "What I see is that functionally, New Hampshire put 90% of its Medicaid program onto the feds instead of 50%. That's why I can live with it" (quoted in Jimenez 1993, NH6).

For hospitals, DSH revenues were a cash bonanza. DSH payments were a classic exercise in distributive politics (Lowi 1969), for while ten institutions received more than $1 million from the program in FY1991 and FY1992, all twenty-seven hospitals were eligible for "enhancement" funds (Jimenez 1992a). With the federal government underwriting a larger share of the state's Medicaid expenditures, program spending ballooned; by 1993, state expenditures on DSH payments were nearly three times those for acute care. Many of the state's hospitals used the additional funds to offset losses from treating Medicaid patients and uncompensated care. The state, for its part, provided hospitals with additional reimbursement with few strings attached in exchange for their endorsement of the gross receipts tax on patient revenues. Although the program dispensed more than $25 million to hospitals in FY1991 and FY1992, the draft rules developed by state officials in the Department of Health and Human Services did not require participating hospitals to document the number of persons served with the additional funds. In defense of the state's hands-off policy, Commissioner Harry Bird contended that "there has to be some sensitivity to the fact that we asked the hospitals for help. All but two of the hospitals are governed by public boards of trustees, many of whom are legislators, so there's a tremendous amount of accountability from that alone" (quoted in Jimenez 1992a, NH17).

Several factors have limited the political appeal of hospital cost containment in New Hampshire over the past decade. On the one hand, the state's health care costs in per capita terms, as well as its supply of hospital beds, remains below average for both the United States and the region. Furthermore, the need for coercive state action to regulate the hospital industry was obviated by the flood of federal funds in the early 1990s. Although Congress significantly tightened the ability of states to reap new revenues from cost-shifting after 1992, New Hampshire's hospital industry remains in reasonably strong fiscal health. Few challenges to the state's market regime loom on the horizon.

HEALTH CARE POLICY-MAKING IN A MARKET REGIME

The politics of health care regulation in New Hampshire reflect the larger political environment in the state. Political life in the Granite State is a testimonial to the continued relevance of Grant McConnell's (1966) description of the "orthodox" tradition in American politics. The orthodox view of interest groups reflects a "deep-seated faith in the virtue of small units of political and social organization. . . . By contrast, government, especially the national government, parties, and 'politics' in general have been deplored as threats to liberty (McConnell 1966, 5)." McConnell's definition captures the essence of political beliefs in the Granite State, where citizens remain highly skeptical of the need for public intervention. As Winters (1985, 280) notes, "In New Hampshire the questioning of the marginal worth of any proposed government action is the general rule. Usually the presumption is that the loss of private action foregone by new public taxation or regulation will be greater than the benefits that might flow from the new or expanded government program."

Participants in the payment process remain uncomfortable with the idea of governmental regulation of the hospital industry. Alongside this fear of government is a strong belief that private solutions will be able to control costs. The director of provider relations for Blue Cross noted, while rate-setting has been discussed in the legislature, "I think we have demonstrated that we're no worse off because we don't have [regulation], but if we go back to [premium] increases in the high teens there'll be more talk about it." The preference of New Hampshire residents for private rather than public solutions reflects a "fundamental suspicion about the ability of politics, once removed from the grass roots of local communities, to express the best of common actions" (Winters 1985, 277). This dread of public power (Morone 1990a) is evident in the words of another senior Blue Cross manager, who argued that "once we let in government, whether it be the federal or state government, then we can look forward to something akin to the problems we're having with Medicare."[5]

Public officials regularly campaign on conservative platforms that emphasize low taxes and a small role for government. In recent years, most successful candidates for state office have taken what Granite State residents have dubbed "the pledge" by refusing to endorse broad-based state taxes to fund expanded educational or social programs.[6] In contrast, political candidates who have endorsed "liberal" policies have fared poorly at the polls and have had little success in persuading legislators to confront the consequences of continued health care inflation. Democratic gubernatorial candidate Deborah Arnesen endorsed a single-payer approach, but lost to Republican Stephen Merrill in 1992. Merrill's ideas on health care reform reflected a vision of limited government that appealed to New Hampshire voters' traditional distrust of government and preference for private solutions to public problems.[7] Merrill proposed an incrementalist agenda that stressed continued efforts by the states to experiment with Medicaid reforms, tax credits to encourage the uninsured to purchase coverage, and the creation of individual "medical IRAs" to control costs. State officials, for their part, expressed skepticism that state government could effectively manage comprehensive health care reform. As Harry Bird, the state's commissioner of Health and Human Services complained, "We're strangling on blue ribbon from commissions. I don't think that government at the state level can do more than nibble at the edges [of the problem]" (quoted in Milne 1992, NH6).

Legislators and voters remain particularly hostile to government solutions that intrude upon the autonomy of state and local governments. These sentiments were particularly evident in 1996, when the state House of Representatives approved a joint resolution urging Congress to abolish the federal Department of Education (HJR 21, Chapter 60 of the Public Laws of 1996) as a result of its "tendency toward direct, federal control . . . which cannot adequately address the needs and

desires of the states and their local communities." Rather than challenging the professional autonomy of health care providers through restrictive rate-setting and capital expenditure controls, state officials in New
Hampshire have adopted a laissez-faire approach to cost containment
which strives to maximize intergovernmental revenue as a means of
subsidizing the rising costs of Medicaid. Furthermore, despite the
state's interest in promoting competition in health care markets through
both CON and managed care, the state has not sought to empower
consumers by mandating the publication of "report cards" that high-
light differences among institutions on the basis of price and quality
of services. This "hands-off" approach to rising health care costs is
particularly evident in the design of the state's certificate-of-need process; even if they were predisposed to do so, state officials possess few
tools to change patterns of hospital investment and slow the prolifera-
tion of expensive new technologies.

New Hampshire's review process for new institutional health care
services has a narrow mandate targeted at inpatient care; as a result,
many projects are exempt from formal review by the HSPRB. As the
New Hampshire Supreme Court declared in 1988, the state's enabling
legislation does not require that a CON be obtained before offering
new outpatient services, for the statute refers only to "'health care
services provided in or through health care facilities or health maintenance organizations" (RSA 151-C:2). The court's decision in *Catholic
Medical Center and Portsmouth Hospital v. Elliot Hospital* argued that the
enabling legislation "reflects a legislative recognition that most medical
procedures performed on an outpatient basis are customarily less difficult and less costly to perform ... and ... do not warrant the extent
of regulation to which inpatient services are subject." The court justified
its decision to uphold the expansion of expanded cardiac catheterization services at a local hospital by appealing to the virtue of the marketplace. In a unanimous opinion, the court suggested that allowing the
hospital to perform outpatient left-heart catheterization (LHCs) served
the state's interest in promoting competition among providers, for
"other Manchester area hospitals, in order to remain competitive, will
be forced to either reduce their prices for catheterization services or
begin performing LHCs on an outpatient basis. Either one of these
choices would serve the pro-competitive aim of RSA chapter 151-C."
In practice, however, since the number of procedures being performed
on an outpatient basis has increased steadily since the 1970s, the restric-
tion of CON review to inpatient facilities and services sharply restricted
both the scope and effectiveness of capital expenditure controls as a
means of containing health care costs in New Hampshire.

New Hampshire's CON program has displayed little interest in circumscribing the autonomy of health care providers. While CON programs in other states have used the application process as a means of increasing access to health care services for the uninsured (Campbell and Fournier 1993; Hackey 1993b), the HSPRB refused to accept the claims of advocates for the elderly and the poor that the board had an obligation to deny CONs to applicants who had not met their "charitable responsibilities" in 1989 and 1991. Although the CON statute requires the HSPRB to consider the "degree to which the proposed project will be accessible to persons who are medically underserviced" (New Hampshire RSA 151C:7), the state had neither standards specifying adequate levels of free care nor a precise definition of free care itself for the board to use in evaluating applications (Jimenez 1991). Board Chairman Leigh Bosse rejected the attorneys' arguments, noting that he "consistently asked them [Women in Search of Hope] to show us how Elliott [Hospital] is deficient in care vis à vis any other New Hampshire hospital and they couldn't do it. . . . I told them to go to the legislature and have them set the standard [they] want[ed] and then we would enforce it" (quoted in Jimenez 1991, 14). In 1991, however, consumer advocacy groups succeeded in using the CON process to force hospitals seeking to expand their services to provide additional free care for the poor over the objections of the HSPRB. With the aid of attorneys from New Hampshire Legal Assistance, a group representing poor women from one of Manchester's least affluent neighborhoods successfully challenged the HSPRB's decision before the state supreme court, leading to agreements by one of the state's largest hospitals to [1] publicize the availability of free care to non-English-speaking residents, [2] increase outreach efforts to local social service agencies, and [3] establish an appeals process for patients who were denied free care (Jimenez 1991, 14).

Private charity, rather than public subsidies, remains the norm for providing free care to indigent patients in New Hampshire. Charity, however, has become expensive for many providers, who have resorted to more aggressive collection techniques in an effort to recover bad debts from patients during the 1990s. Using a little-known state law, hospitals have pursued adult children of patients to assume their parents' debts and placed liens on patients' homes in an effort to control cost shifting of uncompensated care to other payers (Jimenez 1994). Beyond enacting a school-based insurance program, administered by Healthy Kids Corporation, to increase access to health care for poor children, no significant health care access initiatives were considered by the legislature during the flurry of state health policy reforms in 1993 and 1994 (Intergovernmental Health Policy Project 1994). Furthermore, although New Hampshire led the nation in obtaining Medicaid "enhancement" funds from the federal government from 1991 to 1993, aside from the opening of a new clinic to serve poor patients in Manchester (Jimenez 1992b), additional Medicaid revenues were not used to expand access to care through new programs or initiatives. Significantly, the state's Medicaid managed care waiver application did not propose to expand eligibility to uninsured populations (HCFA 1996c).

POLITICAL INSTITUTIONS IN A MARKET REGIME

The structure of New Hampshire's political institutions severely limits the ability of state government to play a proactive role in health care financing. The relative weakness of state government relative to the private sector and the lack of differentiation within the state's legislative and regulatory institutions is a consequence of the shared beliefs in individualism and laissez-faire economic policies held by policymakers and the public. The state's health care bureaucracy is small in size, limiting its capacity to gather information and develop new policies independent of important actors in its environment (principally Blue Cross and Blue Shield of New Hampshire and the New Hampshire Hospital Association). New Hampshire's ability to fund the development of professionalized bureaucratic institutions is also limited by its lopsided revenue structure; in the absence of broad-based state taxes, most services are funded through property taxes, "sin" taxes on cigarettes and liquor, meals taxes, lottery revenues, and user fees.

The legislature, known as the General Court in New Hampshire, is ill-equipped to assume a leadership role on health care policy-making even if its members were predisposed to do so. New Hampshire's legislators are part-time lawmakers who receive little pay for their duties. Members receive $200 per biennium, plus a small per diem stipend for up to fifteen days of the legislative session, and a mileage allowance. Aside from the legislative leaders, members of the house receive no office space or staff support for legislative research (Egbert and Fistek 1993). Furthermore, the legislature is in session only biannually from January to April, and members typically meet only three days each week (Tuesday through Thursday) during the session; staff support is not available to most members when the legislature is not in session. Legislative politics in the Granite State have a unique flavor, for "the size of the institution and its amateur orientation encourages an enormous volume of bills, most of which are either ill-conceived or poorly drafted" (Winters 1985, 285–86). Since legislative service is not a financially attractive proposition for most residents, turnover remains high; during the 1994–96 term, 37.5% of the Senators and 32.5% of the Representatives in the legislature's lower chamber were in their first term.

Legislative politics in New Hampshire have an unwieldy character as a result of the enormous size of the House of Representatives; with 400 members, it is the nation's largest legislative body. The General Court's limitations have frequently been noted by critics, but changes in the composition of the legislature, the length of the legislative session, or members' salaries require a constitutional amendment, which voters have rejected on several occasions in recent decades. As a result, stability, not change, is the norm in the New Hampshire legislature. Peirce's (1976, 325) complaint that "the list of disabilities of this legislature— ranging from the nation's lowest pay to the lack of annual sessions, the high geriatric quotient, and inadequate staff—is staggering." Consensus-building in such an environment is difficult; the size of the chamber was deliberately designed to foster localism.

Both chambers have a large number of standing committees. In the most recent legislative session, the Senate operated with 18 standing committees, while the House had 24; six joint standing committees included members from both chambers of the General Court. Appointments to committees, as well as committee chairmanships, rest in the hands of the President of the Senate and the Speaker of the House. The lack of legislative support staff to assist members in drafting bills and evaluating competing policy proposals magnifies the influence of industry lobbyists. "Legislators quickly learn to rely on lobbyists for needed information. One member asserted that legislators who are doing their jobs seek out lobbyists, and that the others do not" (Egbert and Fistek 1993, 214). Representatives of the health care industry, Blue Cross, and the medical profession were cited as among the most influential groups in the legislature in terms of their perceived influence (Egbert and Fistek 1993).

Democrats have increased their numbers in the Senate in recent years, but the House has been dominated by a conservative Republican majority for decades; during the 1980s, Republicans enjoyed nearly a 3-to-1 majority in the House. Republicans have also controlled the Senate since 1978, when both parties were deadlocked at 12 seats apiece. In 1996, the party solidified its control over both houses of the General Court despite losing the governor's office: Although they lost seats in both chambers, Republicans retained a comfortable working majority in both houses by capturing 15 of the 24 Senate seats and 227 out of 400 House seats.

New Hampshire's governor is the only elected official chosen by statewide balloting, but the governorship is one of the nation's weakest in terms of appointment powers, budgetary control, tenure potential, and veto powers. In large part, the weakness of the governor's office has its roots in the state constitution, which established an elected governor's council comprised of five members elected by district every two years that is empowered to review state contracts and confirm gubernatorial appointees. Furthermore, "most departments remained governed by boards or commissions, minimally responsive to the governor; indeed, most have terms which are not conterminous with his, so that a new governor is encumbered with a whole administrative machinery that can as easily resist his policies as support them" (Peirce 1976, 323). In 1994, the National Governor's Association rated New Hampshire's governorship as the nation's third weakest (after South Carolina and Vermont).

Republicans dominated the governorship during the past decade; until Jeanne Shaheen's victory in 1996, the party had controlled the governor's office continuously since 1982. However, Republican and Democratic candidates for the governor's office have not pursued policy-differentiated campaigns or governing styles. While the Democratic administration of Hugh Gallen from 1978 to 1982 was less controversial (and less colorful) than that of his Republican predecessor, Meldrim Thomson (see Peirce 1976, 334–37), Gallen's fiscal and regulatory policies were not easily distinguished from those of his Republican predecessor or his successor, John Sununu. In 1995, Republican Governor Steve Merrill enjoyed strong approval ratings in public opinion polls, with more than 60% of state residents approving of his performance in office. The Republican Party's success in controlling the legislature and the governor's office is closely tied to the party's continued hostility to broad-based taxes and a firm commitment to economic development, both of which resonate with the state's conservative political culture.

The election of Governor Shaheen, a moderate Democrat, prompted widespread speculation that the state had become more liberal.[8] The new governor, however, won in 1996 on a probusiness, antitax platform, lending credence to former Republican Senator Warren Rudman's observation that "Democrats are essentially where moderate Republicans used to be" (quoted in Harrop 1996). Indeed, Duane Lockard's (1959, 47) observation that "the powers that be in New Hampshire tend to convert all policy to questions of economy in government, for the obvious purpose of keeping taxes down and keeping a tight checkrein on the service and regulatory functions of government" remains as true in the 1990s as it was four decades ago.

Most government agencies in New Hampshire are underfunded, understaffed, and ill-equipped to challenge industry prerogatives. As Peirce (1976, 323) observed, "When any top executives of the state government die or resign, the governor can only offer New England's lowest salaries to any replacement person he selects." New Hampshire ranked dead last among the fifty states in per capita general revenue in 1990, leaving the state little room to make its lackluster state salaries more attractive to potential applicants. Indeed, one of the principal goals of the state's Medicaid managed care waiver application is to upgrade the data processing and policy analysis capabilities of the Department of Health and Human Services, for the department presently lacks both the personnel and the expertise to administer the type of integrated delivery system envisioned in New Hampshire's 1115 waiver proposal. As Egbert and Fistek (1993, 221) note, "State agencies are as much in need of the information gathered by interest groups as legislators. Agencies are therefore subject to capture by interest groups." Legislators and state officials frequently depend on data and testimony provided by the state hospital association or Blue Cross; the state has lagged behind others in the region in developing health databases and comprehensive health plans to guide facilities and service expansion.

TENSIONS WITHIN NEW HAMPSHIRE'S HEALTH POLICY REGIME

Few internal contradictions threaten the stability of New Hampshire's health policy regime in the 1990s. As a result, no underlying shift in the relationship between state government and health care providers is likely for the foreseeable future. Indeed, health care financing in New Hampshire has been remarkably stable since the late 1980s, when rapid growth in Blue Cross premiums led company officials to redefine the terms of their relationship with the New Hampshire Hospital Association. In the absence of a new fiscal crisis for Blue Cross, state officials have few incentives to press for fundamental changes in the state's market-oriented approach to hospital cost control. Fiscal pressures in the late 1980s, however, threatened to weaken the consensus over private, rather than public, solutions to controlling health care costs.

Since New Hampshire's hospitals depend on Blue Cross for nearly a quarter of their operating revenues, the company's generous cost-based reimbursement scheme has long been a prime target for cost shifting. By the end of 1987, however, the company hovered near insolvency. In the face of a $21 million deficit, Blue Cross officials laid off nearly 10% of its work force, changed its senior management team, and won state approval for group rate hikes in excess of 20%.[9] In 1988, an internal Blue Cross report estimated that roughly 30 cents of every dollar in its premiums could be attributed to costs that had been shifted from other payers (Couture 1988).

Prior to 1988, Blue Cross negotiated reimbursement contracts with the state's 27 hospitals through the New Hampshire Hospital Association (NHHA). Initial negotiations between Blue Cross and the NHHA focused on reimbursement for particular diagnoses and utilization review criteria for hospitalized subscribers. However, as one senior Blue Cross executive noted, the results of the preliminary negotiations were "absolutely nonbinding, and they weren't binding until we got to the individual hospitals." From Blue Cross' perspective, this arrangement was wholly unsatisfactory, for the system was heavily biased against the company and in favor of the hospital industry. While agreements could be hammered out with the NHHA, no enforcement mechanism existed to ensure that the association's member hospitals would sign the contract. As one Blue Cross executive recalled, if the hospitals "liked what we talked about and the terms we agreed to, they bought it. If they didn't, they'd say that [the hospital association] was not negotiating for them. Basically, the hospital association, in our opinion, could not deliver the hospitals."

Blue Cross and Blue Shield of New Hampshire, like its counterparts in other states, found itself in a desperate financial predicament as the 1980s drew to a close. Premiums were rising more than 20% annually (Elder 1991), while the company continued to reimburse hospitals on the basis of their charges minus a small (typically 2%) discount. The state insurance commissioner's decision to permit Blue Cross to abandon its traditional method of community-rated premiums—in which all subscribers paid the same rates—to risk-rating on the basis of age and sex was intended to improve the company's weak fiscal position. In response to complaints from consumers over dramatic premium increases, the state's deputy insurance commissioner responded that "we'd love to roll the rates back, but if we did that Blue Cross would be insolvent in a very short period of time" (quoted in Kiernan 1991, 10).

Blue Cross' desperate financial circumstances in the late 1980s was a direct result of its accommodative stance toward providers. As the director of provider relations for Blue Cross explained, the company's individual negotiations with hospitals in the mid-1980s were "based on whether the hospitals had reasonable financial requirements, making it hard to come to an agreement because it was difficult to define [what those were]."[10] Company officials expressed frustration with their lack of credibility and weak bargaining position in negotiations. While the company's average discount was 2%, one Blue Cross executive noted that "some hospitals didn't even send [the contracts] back, and we didn't do anything about it." Blue Cross' lack of credibility could be traced to its subscriber certificate, which laid out the terms of the company's relationships with health care providers and individual subscribers. Prior to 1988, if a hospital did not sign a contract with

Blue Cross, its certificate gave the company two options: it could either pay the hospital 100% of charges or it could pay the subscriber 100% of the charges. Under these circumstances, Blue Cross could neither punish noncompliant hospitals nor encourage its subscribers to use participating institutions. New Hampshire Blue Cross and Blue Shield lived up to its status as a hospital service corporation; under the terms of its subscriber certificate, it had no choice.

This state of affairs changed in 1988, however, when Blue Cross filed a request for an endorsement, or amendment, to its subscriber certificate with the state's insurance department. To win approval of the proposed changes, Blue Cross needed to convince the insurance commissioner that subscribers would benefit under the new system; its argument was that subscribers would reap benefits in the form of lower premiums as a result of the company's improved bargaining position. Blue Cross won its endorsement, but the hospitals failed to realize the effect it would have on them at the time. The amended subscriber certificate allowed the company to refuse to pay benefits to nonparticipating providers; instead, Blue Cross would pay the subscriber 80% of his or her costs, thus creating pressure for individual hospitals to establish contracts with Blue Cross. The change was significant, in the words of one Blue Cross official, because it changed both the direction and the level of reimbursement for hospital services— Blue Cross would no longer recognize nonparticipating providers as legitimate contractual partners. If they failed to sign a contract, hospitals would receive less money from Blue Cross patients, and the patients themselves would have a strong fiscal incentive to seek care at a cooperating institution. In the words of one senior Blue Cross official, "Hospitals couldn't just ignore us anymore, thinking that we'd just go away."

In addition to the new contractual leverage afforded them by the ability to deny contracts to nonparticipating providers, Blue Cross instituted two other significant changes in 1988. First, the company refused to negotiate contracts through the state hospital association; the nonbinding character of the negotiations made participation fruitless from the company's viewpoint. Second, the company ceased its policy of reimbursing providers based on their financial requirements and switched to a price-based system. Under the old system, every hospital had different financial requirements, which led to different prices for the same services at different institutions. The success of individual negotiations, however, was linked to moving to a new basis for reimbursement. Individual negotiations had taken place prior to 1988, but they always focused on the financial requirements of institutions, a process which seldom resulted in consensus. Negotiations based on price were far different, however, for as one Blue Cross official argued, the company was now able to "go to an individual hospital and say 'Here's what your prices are compared to the rest of the world; if you don't negotiate with us, you'll see a significant reduction in your reimbursement.'"[11]

Many hospitals responded to the new Blue Cross policy with disbelief. As one company executive noted, hospital executives "didn't believe that we were going to follow through on [our threat to lower reimbursement] and they called the insurance department to ask if we could do that—they couldn't believe that we were going to do that." Hospitals could be excused for their incredulous reaction, for the company's reputation was not one of strength and conviction. In the end, however, Blue Cross negotiated contracts with all of the state's acute-care hospitals for the 1988–89 fiscal year. As one official recalled, "The first few hospitals went to the eleventh hour before we got a contract, but once the word spread [that we were serious] it's been a pretty smooth process" (Couture 1990). After several years under the new system of individual negotiations with providers over the price of services, Blue Cross has come out a clear winner. The company's average discount off of charges increased from roughly 2% before 1988 to an average of 8 to 9% by the early 1990s. Blue Cross also began to use its market leverage to discourage hospitals from increasing their charges.[12] After 1988, Blue Cross refused to allow hospitals to increase their charges more than 10% in a fiscal year; for every percentage point increase over 10%, the company demanded a commensurate increase in its discount.

Prior to 1988, the NHHA was a major player in the reimbursement process, serving as an intermediary between the hospitals and Blue Cross in contract negotiations. The state's insurance commissioner granted Blue Cross' request, opening the door for Blue Cross to enter into individual negotiations with hospitals. As a result of this arrangement, the New Hampshire Hospital Association became largely irrelevant in the reimbursement decision-making process. After 1988, its role receded from that of a political power broker mediating negotiations to that of an information clearinghouse for member hospitals which provided discharge and expense data to Blue Cross and the state. While these changes left the hospital association out in the cold, relations between the two major players have returned to normalcy. As one Blue Cross executive described it, "We've established a good, solid business relationship [with the hospital association] where we're not just going to roll over and play dead." In part, this may be the result of the hospital association's gradual acceptance of its diminished role in the payment process; since contract negotiations bypass the association, little ground for disagreement between NHHA and Blue Cross officials exists. Barring a return to premium increases at the level of the late 1980s (Elder 1991), neither the hospitals nor Blue Cross are likely to press for significant changes in the state's health care policy regime.

CONCLUSION

The stable operation of a market regime depends upon the maintenance of consensus among the various public and private actors, for actors who operate at a competitive disadvantage under the status quo have an incentive to press for governmental relief. Support for market competition is strong among voters and policymakers in New Hampshire; indeed, the state constitution explicitly endorses competition as a policy goal. As Article 83 of the New Hampshire Constitution declares, "Free and fair competition in the trades and industries is an inherent and essential right of the people and should be protected against all monopolies and conspiracies which tend to destroy it." Instead of regulating providers, the state has sought to increase its leverage as a purchaser of care and encouraged providers to collaborate in order to improve the efficiency of the health care system.

The stability of New Hampshire's market regime has also been reinforced by external changes at the federal level during the 1990s. The infusion of cash from Medicaid disproportionate-share hospital (DSH) payments early in the decade helped to restore the industry to fiscal health. Congressional passage of the Medicaid Voluntary Contribution and Provider Specific Tax Amendments of 1991 and the Omnibus Budget and Reconciliation Act of 1993 limited the state's ability to tap DSH funds to shift additional program costs to the federal government. Nevertheless, the impact on New Hampshire to date has been minimal, for while the 1991 legislation limited state spending on DSH payments to 12% of total Medicaid expenditures, it allowed "high DSH" states such as New Hampshire to continue to provide DSH payments to providers at FY1992 levels. Since New Hampshire's DSH payments actually exceeded Medicaid costs for inpatient hospital care in recent years, the new limitations are unlikely to lead to a rapid rise in state Medicaid costs. In FY1993, DSH payments to state-operated and private hospitals in New Hampshire totaled more than $411 million; the state retained more than $162 million in "residual funds" from the gross receipts tax on providers (Ku and Coughlin 1994, 17).

Furthermore, the implementation of New Hampshire's Section 1115 Medicaid waiver is expected to further reduce pressures on the state budget. Unlike many state waiver applications, New Hampshire will not expand eligibility to uninsured populations or underserved groups; eligibility will be expanded in the future only if "sufficient savings are realized" from the Community Care Systems program. Indeed, the terms of the state's 1115 waiver would effectively insulate New Hampshire from incurring higher than anticipated costs, for the state proposed an aggregate budget cap for the five years of the demonstration from FY1998 through 2002. Finally, since all AFDC-eligible Medicaid patients will be enrolled in the new system, the waiver enhances the state's ability to extract significant cost savings through competitive bidding; under the state's existing Section 1915 waiver, patient enrollment is voluntary and not all areas of the state are served by participating MCOs.

Aside from the enactment of a Medicaid block grant, New Hampshire's health care policy regime remains insulated from policy changes by other actors in its external environment as a consequence of the state's laissez-faire approach to cost containment. Since New Hampshire has not relied upon either state rate-setting, employer-mandated health insurance, or assessments on insurers and providers to fund uncompensated care, it has not run afoul of ERISA's preemption clause. As a result, the role of federal and state courts in New Hampshire is limited to resolving differences between private interests or challenging policymakers' interpretations of the state's limited statutory mandate in CON cases.

Despite the election of the state's first Democratic governor in more than a decade in 1996, major shifts in health care policy are unlikely, for Republicans maintained a stranglehold over both houses of the state legislature and the governor's council. Indeed, although the new governor vowed in her first press conference to make health care more accessible, she forswore the use of broad-based taxes to do so during her campaign (Jacobs 1996). Even if she were predisposed to pursue an activist agenda, however, Shaheen faces staunch opposition from a legislature solidly controlled by conservative Republicans. In the end, few substantial differences exist between the two parties on key taxing and spending issues (Harrop 1996); while Democrats favor more spending on human services and education than their Republican colleagues, Democrats have not advocated a significant increase in public authority to achieve these goals. Instead, Democrats support incremental changes (e.g., state funding for kindergarten) and more local aid than their Republican colleagues.

The diffuse support for market solutions to health care costs in New Hampshire minimizes tensions among public and private participants. As a result, the policy image of health care has not changed appreciably over the past decade. Managed care is changing the nature of the health care industry in New Hampshire as it is elsewhere in the United States, but in recent years hospitals have sought to increase cooperation and resource sharing. The state has encouraged competition among health care providers over the past decade, but not at the expense of forcing institutions to close or change their missions. In 1994, the goals of New Hampshire's CON act were changed by the legislature to reflect this new orientation; the state HSPRB is now directed to promote collaboration, not competition, among providers as a means of controlling costs. Although the state has an excess of hospital beds, officials in the Department of Health and Human Services have allowed hospitals to "swing" beds from acute care to long-term care in order to maintain the viability of many rural hospitals. In short, no crisis in hospital finance or uncompensated care has drawn the attention of legislators or the general public in the 1990s; as a result of their participation in the state's Medicaid revenue enhancement efforts, many hospitals are now in stronger fiscal health than they were a decade ago.

In the absence of compelling fiscal pressures, public officials have little to gain and much to lose by challenging the power of well-financed provider groups. New Hampshire's experience bears this out. Although Medicaid costs are rising rapidly, as in other states, acute hospital care accounts for a relatively small proportion of program expenditures in New Hampshire. Under these circumstances, the development of the institutional and legal authority required to aggressively control hospital costs is difficult to justify in the face of strong resistance to "big government."

CHAPTER NOTES

1. Chapter 391 of the Public Laws of 1983 specified that the HSPRB's membership should include representatives from the departments of health and human services, insurance, and administrative services; five "purchasers or consumers," including at least one representative from the state's business and labor communities; and one representative each from the hospital industry, the nursing home industry, and any other health provider group (New Hampshire RSA 151-C:3). The size of the board was reduced during the 1994 legislative session, and the membership presently includes a representative of the division of public health services, who is the only permanent member of the board; three consumer representatives; two provider representatives nominated by the New Hampshire Hospital Association and the New Hampshire Health Care Association; and a representative from the state's health insurance industry.

2. Prior to 1991, the threshold for CON review of health care facilities' construction, renovation, and expansion projects was $1 million.

3. Appeal of Behavioral Science Institute, NH 436 A.2d 1329.

4. Letter from Arthur Chicaderis, administrator for the Bureau of Program Planning and Policy Development in the New Hampshire Department

of Health and Human Services, to Michelle McEwen, vice president for finance, New Hampshire Hospital Association.

5. In the eyes of the hospital industry, Medicare's unilateral attempt to control its own costs through the implementation of its prospective payment system (PPS) was accompanied by inadequate reimbursement for providers, unstable financial situations even for well-managed institutions, and counter-productive incentives. PPS exacerbated existing trends toward decreasing patients' average length of stay, leading to charges of premature discharges and increased patient mortality, particularly among the elderly. See Lindberg et al. (1988) and Hadley (1988) for evidence supporting these claims.

6. The willingness of 1992 Democratic gubernatorial candidate Deborah Arnesen to consider new broad-based taxes in order to stabilize the state's precarious fiscal situation was widely regarded as one of the principal causes of her electoral defeat.

7. Empirical support for this claim can be found in both survey-based and policy-based measures of state political ideology. Using the measure of state policy liberalism developed by Wright et al. (1985), New Hampshire residents ranked 35th out of the 50 states and the District of Columbia in their aggregate responses to CBS/New York Times polls conducted between 1976 and 1982 (Holbrook-Provow and Poe 1987, 402). New Hampshire's conservatism is also evident in Rosenstone's (1983) concept of New Deal social welfare liberalism and in measures of policy liberalism based on the roll-call voting of state congressional delegations (Holbrook-Provow and Poe 1987).

8. Any notions that the 1996 election marked a turning point in the state's conservative political tradition should be dispelled by the results of other elections for state and national office; Republicans won both seats in the U.S. House of Representatives and a close race for the U.S. Senate.

9. Since the company's unpaid claims exceeded its reserve funds by more than $20 million in 1987–88, senior Blue Cross officials met with staff from the state insurance commission twice weekly to monitor its deteriorating financial situation. At the height of the crisis, Insurance Commissioner Louis Bergeron urged the company to "look at all the possibilities, be it a takeover or a merger or whatever" (United Press International 1988).

10. Under standard hospital accounting procedures, charges represent the financial requirements of the institution, but they often do not correspond with the price of providing a particular set of services. Cost- or charge-based reimbursement makes it difficult for third-party payers to determine a hospital's financial requirements because by definition an institution's financial requirements are what it spent on operations and capital over the course of its fiscal year.

11. When Blue Cross reimbursed hospitals according to their financial requirements, it had to take the overall needs of the institution into account when figuring out its payments, not merely the costs incurred by its patients. The new system of price reimbursement, however, focuses only on Blue Cross patients. Beginning in 1988, Blue Cross used a DRG classification system to compare costs among the state's hospitals. The company establishes its price for each DRG, using Medicare weights to account for differences in the complexity of cases. The price computed for a given treatment in each hospital is

compared to the state average for that procedure, allowing Blue Cross to rank hospitals based on their cost per case. If the state average for a procedure is $1,500, a given hospital's charge might be 110% of that or 90% of that. DRGs are used only for interhospital comparisons, however, not for computing hospitals' rate of payment.

12. Merely increasing the size of Blue Cross' discount is not sufficient for controlling the cost of hospital care nor necessarily even for making the company more profitable. If hospitals can increase their charges at will, Blue Cross would be paying more for the same set of services, even with a larger discount.

7

Rethinking State Health Care Regulation

"Two or three hundred thousand federal employees will regulate every detail of the furnishing of medical service. Certainly nothing could be more intrusive into the freedom of the American family than government medicine of this kind." Senator Robert Taft (R-OH), 1948.

"You can be sure that one day we will awaken to find a bureaucrat sitting alongside us in the consulting room, a politician almost at our elbows in surgery, and government clerks approving or rejecting our prescriptions." Dr. John Galbraith, President, New York State Medical Society, 1962.

"If the [Clinton Health Security Act] passes, you will have to settle for one of the low-budget health plans selected by the government. The law will prevent you from going outside the system to buy basic health coverage you think is better, even after you pay the mandatory premium. The bill guarantees you a package of medical services, but you can't have them unless they are deemed 'necessary' and 'appropriate.' That decision will be made by government, not by you and your doctor." Elizabeth McCaughey, The Manhattan Institute, 1994.

Throughout the 20th century, physicians, hospitals, and conservative politicians have favored private solutions to control rising health care costs and increase access to health care for underserved populations. During this same period, proposals to create a national health insurance system have been assailed by providers on the grounds that it would "regiment" physicians, erode the quality of medical care, and lead to a glut of "red tape." As Senator Orrin Hatch (R-UT) argued in 1992, "I have never heard of any product or service which, if regulated by government, you get better choice, quality, and supply" (quoted in Rovner 1992, 174).

By the mid-1990s, the image painted by opponents of national health insurance had taken shape, as a growing number of hospitals teetered on the brink of fiscal collapse, threatening access to care for residents in both rural communities and inner-city neighborhoods. The clear irony of these developments, of course, is that the deteriorating fiscal health of health care providers and steady erosion of physicians' ability to practice medicine unfettered by "intrusive regulations" in the 1990s was the direct result of intensified market competition, not the introduction of national health insurance. In Germany, Japan, and other nations with universal health insurance programs, health care providers enjoy more professional autonomy than their American counterparts (Wilsford 1995).

Managed care, rather than a federal takeover of medicine, has restructured the U.S. health care system over the past decade, and over the course of two decades the professional autonomy of the medical profession steadily deteriorated in the face of the unrelenting pursuit of cost containment. Physicians must now obtain prior authorization before performing many "overutilized" procedures or referring their patients to specialists. In addition, a growing number of procedures are now performed on an outpatient basis to reduce patients' length of stay and control costs.[1] Furthermore, new "practice standards" have sharply circumscribed physician authority over treatment decisions, which must now be approved by "case managers" employed by managed care organizations (MCOs). To make matters worse, each of these intrusions on the practice of medicine has been accompanied by a growing demand for new data, clinical documentation of treatment decisions for a multitude of payers, and new layers of bureaucracy.

STATE REGULATION AND THE NEW AMERICAN HEALTH CARE SYSTEM

Responsibility for managing these rapid changes in the organization and delivery of health care, however, rests squarely on the shoulders of state governments. Growing competition in the health care industry has changed the role of state governments, reconfigured health care advocacy coalitions and interests, and made existing state policy tools obsolete or less relevant. Increased competition for patients among insurers and the ability of payers to negotiate lower rates for health services with providers operating at less than full capacity led to dramatic savings for employers. After decades of steady inflation, the cost of health benefits declined for the first time in 1994, and rose a meager 2.1% in 1995 after a decade in which double-digit cost increases were commonplace (Pham 1996). Hospital cost increases also moderated in the 1990s (Guterman, Ashby, and Greene 1996; Levit, Lazenby, and Sivarajan 1996). Per capita spending on hospitals rose 3.4% in 1994, compared to 9.6% in 1990 (Ginsberg and Pickreign 1996). While critics regarded the drop in costs as merely the latest example of a "voluntary effort" by the industry to forestall federal and state action, changes elsewhere in the health care system also suggest that managed care has contributed to a fundamental reorganization of health care delivery in the United States. Several state governments reported enormous savings after enrolling millions of eligible Medicaid beneficiaries into managed care plans; early studies of Tennessee's Medicaid managed care program (TennCare) estimated that the implementation of Tenn-Care saved the state more than $1 billion since its inception in 1994 (Brown 1996a; Mirvis et al. 1995).

The decision of many states to embrace managed care as the principal cost-containment strategy, however, creates a dilemma for policymakers. Mandatory enrollment in managed care has the potential to rein in rapidly rising Medicaid costs, but the public remains apprehensive about efforts to reduce subscriber utilization of inpatient hospital care and specialist services as a means of controlling costs. In particular, signs of a public "backlash" against managed care are increasingly evident in the 1990s, as consumers, legislators, and providers seek formal protections for patients (Bodenheimer 1996). Prior to Congressional approval of legislation mandating 48-hour hospital stays for normal vaginal deliveries and 96-hour stays for Cesarean sections, 28 states had passed similar protections for maternity care. Ironically, although third-party payers have traditionally been partners in state efforts to control costs, the growing use of restrictive managed care arrangements by insurers has raised new concerns about the quality of care provided to the elderly, the poor, and patients who require costly treatments (Brown 1996b; Ware et al. 1996). New demands from patients and providers to ensure access to specialists, preserve the professional autonomy of physicians, and establish minimum standards of care for various medical procedures, however, threaten to fracture existing alliances between private third-party payers and state governments. Under these circumstances, what does the future hold for state health care regulation?

With few prospects for enacting comprehensive health care reform at the federal level in the coming decade (Hackey 1993a; Hacker 1996; Steinmo and Watts 1995), responsibility for coping with the dramatic changes in the organization and financing of health care will rest solidly in the hands of state governments (Grogan 1995). Changes in the health care industry will shift the focus of state health care regulation from price-setting and managing the supply of health care facilities and services to quality assurance, consumer protection, and antitrust activities. The policy instruments used by states will change, while many of the essential patterns of regulatory politics described in the preceding chapters will remain. In short, a clear understanding of the factors which contributed to the stability and success of past state cost-containment policies offer the best hope of assessing the problems and prospects of contemporary reforms.

POLICY LESSONS FROM THE NORTHEASTERN STATES AND BEYOND

The regime framework applied in previous chapters informs our understanding of state health care policy-making by emphasizing the interplay of ideas, institutions, and interests in shaping policy. In particular, three features of state health policy regimes will shape state-society relations as public officials continue their efforts to manage changes in the financing and delivery of health care over the next decade. First, the prevailing ideology among public and private elites will play a critical role in both shaping the policy image of health care reform and in defining the range of "legitimate" policy options. Second, the experiences of New York and Massachusetts suggest that internal contradictions within a policy regime can undermine support for regulatory solutions to health care costs over time among payers, providers, and legislators. Finally, each of the case studies discussed in the proceeding chapters suggests that fiscal crises provide state officials with powerful incentives to challenge the prerogatives of health care providers. In the event that market solutions fail to control costs for employers or state Medicaid programs, price regulation is likely to regain legitimacy as a viable policy option.

Ideology and Policy Images

By redefining the range of politically acceptable policy solutions, candidates, elected officials, and policy think tanks will continue to have a powerful impact on state health policy choices in the coming decade. Ideological shifts in Massachusetts and New York laid the groundwork for a fundamental restructuring of state policies toward the health care industry over the past decade. In both states, conservative candidates attacked existing state regulatory controls as inefficient and ineffective. Both William Weld and George Pataki promised to dismantle state rate-setting systems if elected in favor of a market-oriented approach; the discussion of health care financing issues on the campaign trail, in turn, sparked a wider debate over the future of state payment policies among legislators, industry groups, and think tanks. Growing support for deregulating hospital financing in Massachusetts and New York paralleled the ascendance of conservatism within each state's Republican Party; in both states, moderate governors (Ed King and Nelson Rockefeller, respectively) had presided over the creation or expansion of state regulatory controls over the hospital industry. While the hospital payment systems in both states had drawn fire from providers, the antigovernment appeals of conservative gubernatorial candidates provided a rallying cry for proponents of deregulation. The power of ideology to transform a state's health policy agenda is particularly evident in light of this experience, for less than a year after electing conservative Republican governors, two of the nation's most heavily regulated hospital payment systems had embraced market competition and renounced the rate-setting programs each had pioneered more than a decade earlier.

The impact of changes in ideology on policy is particularly salient in light of proposals by Republicans in the 104th Congress and the National Governors' Association to devolve more policy-making responsibilities over health care issues to state governments. A recent review of gubernatorial policy agendas by Daniel Dileo (1996) suggests that the devolution of health care policy-making for Medicaid to the states would have significant policy repercussions at the state level for poor and underserved populations. Although most governors routinely espouse support for expanded access to care and more aggressive efforts to control costs, governors expressed less support for redistributive policies to improve access to care for the poor than either George Bush or Bill Clinton. Indeed, the policy image of state regulatory efforts has changed following the demise of the Clinton administration's ill-fated health care reform package. Significantly, however, the policy image of state hospital regulation changed in Massachusetts and New York prior to legislators' decision to deregulate each state's hospital payment system. At the time regulatory controls expired in both states, rate-setting was no longer seen as a solution to controlling health care costs, but as a cumbersome and outdated burden on hospitals and third-party payers.

In an ironic twist, managed care, once the solution to the health care system's woes espoused by many conservative reformers, itself became a policy problem. Since 1995, the rapid growth of managed care plans redefined prevailing notions of market competition in the health sector among policymakers and the public. New "casual stories" (Stone 1988) emphasized managed care abuses, focusing attention on the use of financial incentives to reward physicians who relied less on high-cost procedures and specialist referrals and "gag clauses" that precluded doctors from informing their patients of treatment options not covered by their health plan. By the mid-1990s MCOs were increasingly cast in a negative light as faceless, profit-maximizing bureaucracies that routinely placed the pursuit of profit above concerns for patient welfare.[2] HMO-bashing soon crossed partisan and ideological boundaries as a "safe" issue that was popular with voters. As the *New England Journal of Medicine* editorialized, "The quality of health care is now seriously threatened by our rapid shift to managed care as the way to control costs" (quoted in Pear 1996). In response to this threat, governors and states legislatures across the United States appointed study commissions, held hearings, and introduced a flurry of legislation designed to protect patients from abuses by MCOs.

Internal Contradictions

The experiences of Massachusetts and New York also illustrate how changing group interests and market forces can undermine the stability of a policy regime. These causal agents varied from state to state, but in each case a growing incompatibility emerged between the existing system of regulatory controls and the interests of key public and private actors in the regime. In Massachusetts, support for rate-setting by business groups evaporated in the wake of numerous concessions to providers required to win legislative passage of the state's universal health care law. After 1988, business leaders lost faith in the political process as a means of controlling employee health care costs; in lieu of system-level cost containment, firms increasingly turned to benefits management and managed care as their principal cost-control strategy.

In New York, several factors conspired to undermine a political coalition in support of rate-setting that had survived for more than two decades. On the one hand, as the state's enrollment in managed care plans increased in the early 1990s, third-party payers sought the ability to bargain for volume discounts with providers. Providers, for their part, had successfully challenged the surcharges embedded in the state's prospective reimbursement methodology (NYPHRM) in both state and federal courts on the grounds that it violated the Employee Retirement and Income Security Act of 1974 (ERISA). Although New York's rate-setting program survived its legal challenge on appeal to the U. S. Supreme Court, in the absence of strong support from third-party payers, legislators began to explore alternative policy instruments which could accommodate the divergent interests of providers, payers, and the state.

Fiscal Crisis

In both Massachusetts and New York, fiscal crises preceded dramatic shifts in state policy toward the health care industry. The rhetoric of crisis, whether perceived or actual, can break down traditional relationships between interest groups and the state and, in the process, can legitimate previously unthinkable policy choices. Fiscal crises, however, can also facilitate the creation of an imposed regulatory regime. The swift creation and implementation of TennCare in 1994 suggests that the policy lessons from the Northeastern states are paralleled elsewhere. In Tennessee, legislators granted Democratic Governor Ned McWherter unprecedented authority to reengineer the state's health care financing system in the wake of a budget-busting Medicaid shortfall and a rapid growth in Medicaid enrollment. Medicaid spending in Tennessee quadrupled from FY1989 to FY1994, consuming nearly one-quarter of the state's budget in 1993 (Brown 1996a; Mirvis et al. 1995). As the governor warned state legislators in 1993, "No issue is more urgent, and without a solution, the entire state government in Tennessee remains in jeopardy" (quoted in Brown 1996a). McWherter's solution to the state's fiscal crisis was TennCare, a mandatory Medicaid managed care demonstration program designed to improve the managerial efficiency of health care for the poor and uninsured while controlling costs through a heavily discounted fee-for-service reimbursement methodology.

TennCare created a managed care industry in Tennessee almost overnight, for the state was determined to implement the program within a single year after its passage. As Meyer and Blumenthal (1996) observed, the rapid pace of implementation under the threat of fiscal catastrophe provided state officials with a crucial advantage in negotiating with providers, payers, and advocates for the poor, for administrative chaos accompanying the short implementation timetable made it difficult for stakeholders to organize a campaign to repeal or postpone the principal features of the plan.[3] Although perceptions of an emerging crisis led to the adoption of Medicaid managed care plans in Massachusetts, New York, and Tennessee in the 1990s, previous fiscal crises paved the way for the creation of state rate-setting programs in the 1970s and 1980s. In short, while the exact nature of a state's response to a fiscal crisis will reflect the prevailing policy images of potential solutions and the ideological tenor of the times, crises provide public officials with a unique opportunity to advance the state's interests in the face of significant societal resistance.

POLICY REGIMES IN A COMPETITIVE MARKETPLACE

Although a majority of states have now embraced managed care as a primary cost-control strategy, the nature and form of "procompetitive" strategies vary widely from state to state. In short, different policy regimes craft dissimilar strategies to harness market forces, and conversely, to protect patients and consumers from the vagaries of the market. Indeed, both the active efforts of public officials to nurture competition among providers and payers and policies to cushion patients and providers from "destructive" competition are measures of state strength in a competitive marketplace. By establishing ground rules for competition, or mitigating its effects on vulnerable populations, states can harness markets as a policy tool to achieve public purposes (Schultze 1977). In an era of growing competition among payers and providers, distinctions between imposed, negotiated, and market regimes reflect the extent to which government officials adopt a proactive—as opposed to reactive—stance towards "managing" competition to achieve the state's interests.

Under an imposed regime, the state actively promotes competition as a means of controlling costs and increasing access to care in the face of opposition from providers or payers. Medicaid managed care waivers, for example, can be used to significantly expand access to care for persons without health insurance by plowing cost savings from capitation for program enrollees into state-subsidized insurance programs for the working poor. States can also impose a mandatory budget cap on regional or statewide health care expenditures, forcing providers to compete for a share of a fixed pool of funds allocated by a health care authority or purchasing cooperative. In both cases, state officials are not merely passive observers of market competition but instead channel and direct market forces in pursuit of public purposes (e.g., controlling Medicaid costs). Imposed regimes, however, will be characterized by a state-led switch to market mechanisms as a means of achieving the state's own goals, rather than reacting to the concerns of providers, payers, or other societal interests.

Tennessee's embrace of managed care for Medicaid beneficiaries offers the most striking example of how an imposed regime can emerge in a competitive health care system, for the introduction of TennCare "transformed the provision of health care to Medicaid beneficiaries from a seller's market into a buyer's market" (Bonneyman 1996, 306). The creation of TennCare was a calculated response to an emerging fiscal crisis, for the governor exploited the chaotic atmosphere to reduce Medicaid payments to providers, expand the scope of state authority over health care reimbursement, and force a wholesale reorganization of health care delivery upon providers (Mirvis et al. 1995). The state was an unlikely candidate to embrace managed care as its principal cost-control strategy, for Tennessee had high health care costs, low managed care penetration, and few managed care providers offering services throughout the state. Prior to 1993, only 6% of the state's population was enrolled in any form of managed care plan (Brown 1996a). Providers initially balked at TennCare's capitation rates, as primary care physicians, academic medical centers, community health centers, and specialists claimed that the state's capitation rates were unreasonably low. During its first year, TennCare survived a "walkout" by nearly a third of all participating Blue Cross physicians and scathing studies by the Tennessee Hospital Association and the legislature's own oversight committee that indicated that the program paid hospitals slightly more than 50% of their actual costs for patient care, forcing institutions to cost-shift to other payers (Meyer and Blumenthal 1996). As such, the enactment and implementation of the state's Medicaid waiver represented a fundamental realignment of purchasing power within Tennessee's health policy regime.

In other states, the design of regulatory controls allows rate-setting to coexist as a complementary cost-containment strategy to competitive bidding among HMOs for health care services. As Maryland's experience over the past decade demonstrated, all-payer rate-setting systems are not antithetical to a competitive environment in health care. By using disaggregated units of payment and provider-specific conversion factors, Maryland's rate-setting methodology enables MCOs to limit the volume of services provided to patients and to selectively contract with low-cost providers (Wallack et al. 1996). Indeed, various proposals to implement "managed competition" at the state level in the mid-1990s were based upon the notion that price competition among health plans offering a standard benefits package under an aggregate budget constraint offered the best prospect of controlling costs and increasing access to care for the uninsured (Starr and Zelman 1993). As Wilsford (1995, 607) notes in his study of health policies in advanced industrialized nations, "States may even act more dynamically to change the terms through which policy outcomes are collectively decided, sometimes even against entrenched societal interests, as long as the policy imperatives are fairly powerful, such as the fiscal imperative we observe everywhere in health care."

Negotiated regimes are characterized by collaborative problem-solving among public and private actors rather than by confrontation and conflict over policy goals. Affected interests frequently disagree over the proper means of achieving a policy, but key participants hammer out agreements on the principal ends of a policy in private negotiations. Under these circumstances, proposed reforms must offer inducements to win the support of private groups. While such arrangements were particularly evident in health care policy-making in Massachusetts and Rhode Island over the past two decades, negotiated regimes have also emerged in such diverse states as Florida, New York, and Oregon in recent years.

The creation of public-private partnerships to control costs is a hallmark of negotiated regimes, as state officials enlist the support of businesses and other payers to pool their purchasing power. As Hanson

(1994, 56) notes, health care policy-making in Florida is best described as a negotiated regime, for disagreements among key interest groups provided Governor Lawton Chiles with an opportunity to use the prospect of radical, comprehensive reforms to prod advocates for the elderly, nonprofit hospitals, and for-profit providers to accept a compromise. The state has also taken an active role in stimulating price competition among MCOs by creating a network of community health purchasing alliances (CHPAs) to enable small businesses to purchase competitively priced health insurance. By June 1996, more than 76,000 residents had purchased insurance from one of nine regional alliances funded by the state. Furthermore, Florida has actively embraced managed care for Medicaid beneficiaries by enrolling more than 380,000 persons in HMOs; an additional 600,000 are enrolled in the state's primary care case management program (Demkovich 1996c).

The transformation of New York's imposed regulatory regime is particularly evident in the state's approach to regulating the behavior of MCOs. Indeed, health care policy-making in the Empire State in the mid-1990s is best described as a negotiated policy regime, for state officials have teamed up with providers and payers in pursuit of mutually acceptable policy options. At the same time it deregulated its health care financing system, New York Governor George Pataki signed a sweeping package of legislative reforms designed to protect patients from potential abuses by MCOs. In a departure from the state's authoritative stance toward providers, the legislation was drafted in close consultation with hospitals, physicians, payers, and businesses. The governor's plan aimed to protect patients by (1) barring MCOs from employing physician "gag clauses"; (2) requiring plans to maintain an "adequate network" of participating providers; and (3) mandating that MCOs provide their members with information on covered procedures, billing, and grievance processes to certify specialty MCOs to provide care for persons with HIV.[4] Although New York's actions were among the toughest in the nation, the new policy was widely supported by providers, payers, and consumer groups.

In Rhode Island, the state's negotiated policy regime recently endorsed a series of reforms aimed at protecting consumers from health plan abuses. In the closing days of an extended legislative session marked by acrimonious debates between Governor Lincoln Almond and the General Assembly over the state budget, policymakers ratified the report of a broad-based study commission created by the legislature. The Health Care Accessibility and Quality Assurance Act (96-H-8172) prohibited the use of gag clauses and financial incentives to deny patients care, established a certification process for all MCOs operating in the state, and protected physicians from dismissal by HMOs without cause. As is evident from the preceding cases, negotiated policy regimes have employed a wide range of policy instruments to "manage" competition in the marketplace, from the establishment of purchasing cooperatives to the development of rules governing fair competition among providers and payers. In each case, however, affected interests were directly incorporated into the policy-making process; extensive consultation with industry groups, rather than confrontation, remains a hallmark of negotiated regimes in a competitive market environment. In each case, however, state officials played a prominent, if not vital role, in shaping coalitions for reform and defining the issue agenda to serve public purposes.

Market regimes, in contrast, reflect an enduring belief in the ability of private groups to solve public problems with little or no direct involvement by the state. Under these circumstances, policymakers are prone to "let the market work" with only limited regulation by the state to protect the health and safety of consumers. Indeed, private firms and independent organizations are already driving system change even in the absence of state or federal action. Major employers have spearheaded efforts to create standardized benchmarks for health plans and hospitals in recent years through the Health Plan Employer Data and Information Set (HEDIS) and other local initiatives (Harris 1994a, 1994b). HEDIS, along with the National Committee for Quality Assurance's (NCQA) accreditation program, is designed to offer employers and consumers the ability to compare the performance of health plans in terms of patient satisfaction, the cost of care, access to needed services, the use of preventive services, and clinical outcomes (NCQA 1996). In addition, both the public and private sectors can encourage the development of standardized benefits packages to promote price competition among comparable plans and the dissemination of standardized information on the quality of health services offered by all providers (Enthoven and Singer 1996).

For believers in market solutions, the current wave of mergers and acquisitions in the health care system represents a natural response of providers to intensified competition. In this view, vertical and horizontal integration offers a means to wring excess capacity from the health care system and bring purchasers more "value" for their money by increasing the efficiency of hospital operations. By consolidating legal services, personnel, purchasing, pharmacy, and other management functions, proponents of integration in the health care system argue, new networks or partnerships are able to offer higher-quality services with fewer overhead costs. In addition, proponents of competition argue that hospitals and other health care providers have introduced new "patient management" techniques to reduce the unnecessary utilization of tests, procedures, and hospitalizations. As an example, the growing use of "critical pathways" and other computer-assisted utilization management techniques is designed to create "lanes and barriers" for physicians as they order tests and procedures for patients (Foreman and McClennan 1996). The end result of both external forces (e.g., mergers and consolidations) and internal management changes (e.g., continuous quality improvement techniques and utilization management tools) is expected to be leaner and more efficient providers, with no direct intervention from government.

Market competition has also been hailed as a means to increase the quality of patient care. In contrast to negotiated or imposed regimes, however, market regimes frequently rely upon private organizations to develop rules for their members. In this view, standard-setting can be effectively delegated to professional associations whose concern for the autonomy and economic well-being of their members will encourage the development of voluntary guidelines which will be adopted as de facto norms by providers and payers without the heavy hand of government regulation. As a case in point, new guidelines issued by the American Association of Health Plans (AAHP) are designed to preempt federal or state restrictions on the activities of managed care providers by demonstrating that the marketplace can police itself. The AAHP's policy statement urges its member organizations to provide subscribers with information on how plan physicians are paid, how plans determine which treatments are "necessary," "appropriate," or "experimental" in nature, and to disclose which services or treatments are most appropriate for the patient's condition, regardless of whether they are covered by the plan (*Washington Post* 1996).

THE FUTURE OF STATE HEALTH CARE REGULATION

At century's end, state governments face a new set of challenges in shaping health care policy in a competitive market environment. Rather than setting prices and controlling the diffusion of capital projects, state regulation in the 1990s is increasingly focused on policies to buffer the impact of market forces on vulnerable institutions and populations. In short, the "coming of the corporation" (Starr 1982) has created new needs for state governments to address the negative externalities which accompany the expansion of price competition among providers and MCOs. Although the paths followed by states in softening the impact of market changes will be shaped by the nature of their policy regimes, several emerging areas of health care regulation will occupy a growing share of policymakers' attention in the years to come. First, state governments have recently begun to legislate patterns of medical practice for maternity care, and policymakers have shown interest in establishing minimum hospital stays for other procedures (e.g., mastectomies). Second, state health departments, along with private sector accrediting agencies and third-party payers, have shown tremendous interest in establishing quality benchmarks for providers to better assess the value of health care services purchased on behalf of clients and subscribers. Finally, states continue to have a significant role in ensuring access to care for the uninsured and in maintaining the fiscal health of "essential" community providers in an increasingly competitive health care marketplace.

Setting Standards

One role for state governments in a competitive health care system is to establish rules to protect patients and providers from unfair competitive practices. In 1996, state and federal governments significantly increased their regulation of medical practice by legislating practice standards for certain high-visibility procedures such as maternity care and by limiting the managerial autonomy of MCOs. Regulations governing the length of hospital stays, however, are merely a harbinger of things to come, for as reviews of recent state legislation to regulate the managed care industry by Hellinger (1996) and Bodenheimer (1996) demonstrate, a growing backlash against perceived abuses by MCOs has generated a torrent of new legislation. Across the U. S., states have moved aggressively to prohibit "gag clauses," protect physicians from dismissal by an HMO without "just cause," expand the rights of patients to appeal denials of payment or treatment, and prohibit exclusive contracts between providers and MCOs. The promulgation of new standards of patient care, however, need not occur through legislation, for medical specialties (such as those represented by the American Academy of Pediatrics and the American College of Surgery's Committee on Trauma) have developed voluntary certification programs and recommended treatment protocols for decades.

Efforts by state governments to regulate the delivery of health care services are fraught with difficulty for the agencies charged with monitoring the appropriateness and quality of clinical treatments. In market regimes, standard-setting will typically be implemented through an informal process of professional education conducted by providers themselves through existing professional organizations. Numerous precedents exist for this approach, for professional societies routinely establish treatment protocols for cardiac surgery, trauma care, and other procedures which specify optimal care for patients; establish protocols for clinical appropriateness; and provide criteria for assessing the quality of health care facilities and the training of personnel.[5] State legislation that requires providers to meet the minimum criteria established by professional societies in order to offer specialty services is cost effective and entails a minimal resource commitment on the part of state regulatory agencies. Since such efforts cede responsibility for standard-setting and monitoring to organizations created and staffed by health care providers (e.g., the Joint Commission on the Accreditation of Health Care Organizations), states which adopt this approach to improving the quality of patient services are limited in their ability to set standards more stringent than those established by national organizations or accrediting bodies. In addition, when responsibility for assessing and monitoring the quality of care rests solely in the hands of provider-sponsored organizations, states may find it difficult to obtain independent assessments of provider performance.[6]

As New York demonstrated in the late 1980s, states can impose stringent new quality standards upon the health care industry, but the political costs of such interventions may be too high. Under the leadership of David Axelrod, the state Department of Health developed new regulations (known as "Part 405") to limit the number of hours residents, interns, and fellows could work; establish new emergency department standards; and require that postgraduate trainees be supervised by experienced board-certified (or eligible) physicians. Since the new regulations effectively required hospitals to hire additional staff or upgrade the qualifications of existing staff, the state's efforts were challenged in court by the state hospital association and several of its members. The cost of implementing new standards in the face of concerted opposition from health care providers, as well as the commitment of political and fiscal capital necessary to gather data, monitor compliance, and sanction noncompliant institutions are also high, making such a direct strategy of confrontation unappealing to policymakers.

Furthermore, expanded state regulation of operating conditions and medical practice raises several important questions about enforcement. Will states ban noncompliant providers from participating in the Medicaid program? Impose fines on poor performers? Revoke the operating licenses of institutions with severe deficiencies? Or will state officials publicize the nature and extent of quality problems in hospitals to inform patients and the public? Since hospitals depend on their reputations to attract patients and physicians, negative publicity could adversely affect weaker institutions by leading to a mass exodus to other facilities. In a free market, such an outcome would be viewed as "efficient" by rewarding providers that deliver higher-quality services at a lower cost. However, efforts to improve the quality of care could wreak havoc on the fiscal health of hospitals that disproportionately service low-income and vulnerable (e.g., unprofitable) populations.

The movement toward establishing "rules of the game" for market competition raises two key questions for state health care regulation. Who will establish practice standards and which organizations will accredit and monitor the quality of patient care? At present, the U.S. health care system relies upon an amalgam of public and private accreditation processes. While hospitals and other health care providers (including HMOs) are typically licensed by the state, government agencies routinely rely upon provider-dominated organizations such as the College of American Pathologists to assess the quality of health care services provided by individual institutions and to identify any deficiencies (Hackey and Williams 1996). As providers scramble to cut costs in a competitive marketplace, expanded state quality assurance activities and oversight will be required to protect patients from incentives to provide fewer services, reduce staffing levels, or substitute lower-cost allied health professionals such as certified nurse assistants for more expensive health care personnel. In addition, state efforts to establish patterns of medical practice, as in the case of legislation mandating minimum hospital stays for maternity care, create a number of difficulties for policymakers. If states elect to regulate lengths of stay or treatment options only on an ad hoc basis, the influence and organization of advocacy coalitions of patients and providers will determine which procedures or specialties will be afforded legislative protection. Policymakers in Florida and several other states, however, have embraced a more comprehensive approach to standard-setting by mandating the development of practice guidelines as a means of controlling costs and improving the quality of medical care (Szabo 1995).

A renewed emphasis on the assessment of patient outcomes also points to new roles for state CON programs over the next decade. Recent studies of the appropriate utilization of cardiac catheterizations, coronary angioplasties, and other specialized diagnostic and therapeutic procedures in recent years is driven, at least in part, by reimbursement, for the type of health insurance a patient has is strongly associated with their utilization of health services. In addition, recent studies of these surgical procedures found that many surgical procedures were either "inappropriate" or of "uncertain" clinical value (Grayboys et al. 1992; Chassin et al. 1987b). Although health planners' initial definition of the "need" for new facilities was often vague and imprecise, the growing literature on the appropriate utilization of health services offers regulators concrete clinical standards with which to evaluate applications.

Using recent studies as a benchmark, state regulators are already beginning to apply the guidelines developed by outcomes researchers in evaluating CON applications based on the appropriate utilization of existing services. Legislators in Oregon, for example, linked the approval of new capital projects to an institution's patient outcomes; institutions must demonstrate sufficient patient volume for proposed services, so that "if a new transplant center is proposed, or if a medical facility wants to buy magnetic resonance imaging equipment, questions will be asked about whether the patient base will support it, and whether its purchase will affect patient outcomes" (Alter and Holtzman 1992, 20). In the absence of evidence that proposed services have a significant impact on patient outcomes, the CON process may be used to identify potentially unnecessary facilities and discourage the over-utilization of specialized procedures.

Implementing Quality Assurance

State efforts to improve the quality of patient care have come to the forefront of health care policy-making in recent years. A growing body of empirical evidence indicates that patterns of medical practice, the cost of medical procedures, and patient outcomes differ widely both within and across states. Furthermore, as John Wennberg, John Ware, and others have demonstrated over the past two decades, enormous variations in medical practice did not lead to corresponding differences in patient outcomes (Banham 1992). In response, several states have heeded Paul Ellwood's call for a "public accounting system for health care" by establishing reporting systems to document regional and inter-state variations in treatments, costs, and outcomes. Another key role for state regulation in a competitive health care system lies in developing technology assessment protocols to aid third-party payers, consumers, and businesses in purchasing decisions (Mendelson, Abramson, and Rubin 1995). By evaluating emerging technologies and therapeutic interventions, states may promote the cost-effective use of medical resources.

By 1995, twelve states had enacted legislation that regulated the development or dissemination of clinical practice guidelines, while other states collected and disseminated data on the cost and quality of certain medical procedures. In particular, several state health departments have published "report cards" for hospitals and surgeons for cardiac surgery to assist patients and third-party payers in purchasing cost-effective, high-quality health care services (Pennsylvania Health Care Cost Containment Council 1992). In New York, a cardiac care advisory committee comprised of physicians, hospital representatives, and independent policy think tanks established statewide standards of care for cardiac procedures. The New York State Department of Health gathers data from all health care facilities in its SPARCS dataset and publishes annual reports on costs and patient outcomes to assist hospitals in identifying potential quality problems (New York State Department of Health 1995a). In addition, the state contracted with the RAND Corporation to study the appropriate utilization of cardiac surgery in New York in 1990 (Leape et al. 1993; Hilborne et al. 1993). The state's quality monitoring efforts have won accolades from both providers and payers, as risk-adjusted mortality for cardiac surgery in New York State declined by more than 40% since 1990.

Critics of this approach, however, contend that increasing the availability of information for consumers, monitoring providers, and establishing practice standards are ineffective restraints on the behavior of providers and payers. Marc Rodwin (1996) suggests that organized consumer advocacy groups are needed to demand accountability from MCOs. One option to increase the accountability of providers would be for states to formally incorporate patient advocacy groups within state government. By establishing offices of "patients' rights" or "health care assistance" within state health or insurance departments, policymakers could institutionalize ombudsman services for patients. The creation of health care advocacy groups within state government would empower consumers by encouraging "fair" competition among providers and payers.[7] As Rodwin (1996, 116) notes, "Our system lacks strong institutions or groups that advocate more generally for medical consumers or that can serve subscribers within their own managed care organizations." Alternatively, states could mandate that consumers be provided with strong representation on the governing boards of state-sponsored purchasing cooperatives and health alliances. The latter approach, however, runs the risk of replaying the struggles over representation in the federal health planning program documented by Marmor and Morone (1981), for the simple inclusion of nonproviders in the decision-making process offers few guarantees that consumer interests will be effectively articulated.

Preserving and Enhancing Access to Health Care

By the early 1990s, the health policy agenda had changed; while controlling costs remained the central goal of both state and federal policymakers, the growing number of persons without health insurance and mounting fiscal losses from uncompensated hospital care brought concerns about access to health care back to the health policy agenda. State regulation to ensure access to health care will become increasingly important in the coming decade, for increased market competition threatens the fiscal health of many community hospitals and urban teaching institutions. States face several challenges in ensuring continued access to health care. First, state financing of charity care has come under fire in Florida, Massachusetts, and New York as either inadequate or inequitable.[8] Second, the growing wave of consolidation within the health care industry raises new concerns about access to care for insured and uninsured populations alike, for the service cutbacks or hospital closures that often accompany mergers can make it more difficult for underserved populations to reach health care providers. The expansion of for-profit hospital chains into new markets has raised concerns among providers and policymakers over the provision of charity care to the poor and uninsured. Finally, the growing popularity of Medicaid managed care plans as a means of controlling costs has raised new concerns among advocates for the poor. Since capitation rates for state Medicaid programs are typically set below the rates paid by private insurers, MCOs that enroll a disproportionate number of poor patients may face a strong incentive to provide fewer specialty services to their subscribers.

The problem of uncompensated care appears to be worsening in the 1990s as employers continue to pass along more costs to their workers and/or cut benefits altogether (Weissman 1996). More than 41 million Americans were uninsured in 1995, an increase of more than 5 million since the beginning of the decade. The number of Americans without health insurance is likely to increase for the remainder of the decade despite state initiatives to expand Medicaid eligibility, for the growing use of part-time or temporary workers permits employers to offer insurance to fewer workers. The simultaneous growth of managed care enrollment and the uninsured creates a fiscal bind for hospitals, which face the prospect of treating more patients who cannot pay without the ability to cost shift to charge-based payers. In Florida, for example, the ability of hospitals to fund indigent care through cost shifting was limited by extensive HMO market penetration, an above-average number of for-profit hospitals, and Medicare's status as the largest third-party payer in the state. Confronted by a growing indigent care problem and restrictive Medicaid eligibility requirements, public officials in Florida used their regulatory mandate under the state's CON program to encourage hospitals to provide care for the uninsured (Campbell and Fournier 1993).

Additional threats to the ability of hospitals to provide uncompensated care to a growing population of uninsured patients lurk on the horizon. Bruce Vladek, the Director of HCFA, is now seeking discounts for Medicare similar to those hospitals grant private employers and MCOs (Wessel 1996). In the absence of supplemental reimbursement from either state or federal payers, the most likely outcome of "prudent purchasing" on the part of MCOs, Medicaid, and Medicare is a growing number of hospital closures, reduced patient services, and more mergers and affiliations as weak hospitals seek more profitable partners in order to survive. The deregulation of state rate-setting systems also raises new concerns for hospitals that have an unfavorable case mix of uninsured patients and publicly insured patients. In the past, rate-setting systems in New York and other states assessed a surcharge on hospital charges to fund uncompensated care pools that were distributed among institutions on the basis of need. In the wake of deregulation, the adequacy of state funding of uncompensated care and subsidies for graduate medical education (GME) now presents many urban teaching institutions with a double-edged fiscal threat. While teaching hospitals in New York State are now guaranteed funding for training new physicians through the state's rate-setting methodology, under the state's new deregulated reimbursement system providers will be required to negotiate with third-party payers to fund GME. New Jersey's experience serves as a warning for other states, for nearly five years after the demise of the state's all-payer rate-setting system, state officials have struggled to find a stable financing mechanism for uncompensated care, even as the number of persons without insurance in the state continued to grow (Demkovich 1996a).

The 1990s have also witnessed a surge in merger activity among both for-profit and nonprofit hospitals. By the end of 1996, more than 100 government-owned or nonprofit community hospitals had affiliated with a for-profit health care corporation (Langley and Sharpe 1996). In 1996 alone, 1 in 12 hospitals was involved in a merger or acquisition; more than 450 hospitals merged with major health care holding companies (Demkovich 1996d). The acquisition of nonprofit community hospitals by large proprietary hospital chains such as Columbia/HCA Healthcare Corp. and Tenet Healthcare Corp. has sparked fears that for-profit holding companies would reduce the amount of free care after acquiring community hospitals (Jones 1996). Representative Pete Stark (D-CA) accused Columbia and other for-profit chains of acting as "carpetbaggers" who "have a history of closing local hospitals, creating monopolies, and laying people off" (quoted in Langley and Sharpe 1996). In addition, price competition among MCOs and integrated delivery systems may subside in the future, leading to new antitrust concerns about price-fixing and other collusive behaviors among an oligopoly of health care providers within a state or region (Sage 1996).

As Jack Zwanziger (1995, 172) notes, state antitrust enforcement efforts in the health sector must "prevent the creation of entities that are not constrained by market forces while allowing rationalization and consolidation." In addition, the conversion of several Blue Cross and Blue Shield plans to for-profit status raises important redistributive issues for state health care reimbursement systems. On the one hand, such conversions remove an important safety valve in health insurance markets, for Blue Cross plans typically accept more high-risk (e.g., sicker and less profitable) patients than other health insurers to fulfill their "charitable mission" as nonprofit insurers. In addition, the privatization of Blue Cross plans may disrupt existing relationships among providers and third-party payers in health policy regimes where the dominant organizations have been nonprofit entities.

Several policy instruments are available for states to ensure that the current "merger mania" does not stifle competition among providers, diminish access to care, or compromise the fiscal health of nonprofit institutions. Since many mergers in recent years were negotiated in private with little public input, California enacted legislation in 1996 that required public hearings whenever a for-profit corporation proposes to merge with or acquire a nonprofit hospital (Langley and Sharpe 1996). Elsewhere, state attorney generals have filed suit to block proposed acquisitions by for-profit chains (Demkovich 1996d). In Massachusetts, Attorney General Scott Harshbarger exacted concessions from Columbia/HCA during negotiations over the state's first for-profit merger with a nonprofit community hospital in which Columbia agreed to continue to provide around-the-clock emergency care and maintain the facility's commitment to charity care. States also face a daunting problem in appraising the assets of nonprofit organizations, for corporations such as Columbia/HCA maintain that the disclosure of detailed financial information about proposed mergers would force companies to release privileged trade secrets that would place them at a competitive disadvantage. Nevertheless, states will be increasingly forced to assess the impact of hospital mergers on competition, conduct independent audits of the assets of nonprofit institutions, negotiate the transfer of "charitable assets" from nonprofit entities to independent foundations, and buffer the impact of competition on existing nonprofit providers serving vulnerable populations.

The new health care marketplace brings different challenges for state governments. Daily life in a typical state regulatory agency has changed dramatically since the 1970s and early 1980s, when policymakers invested regulatory agencies with the responsibility to impose rationality on the health care system through areawide planning programs, rate-setting, certificate-of-need controls, and targeted manpower policies. In earlier eras, data collection, citizen involvement, and statistical models to determine the "need" for new facilities and evaluate the "appropriate utilization" of health care services were thought to hold the key to controlling costs. Once in place, however, regulatory controls often proved to be cumbersome, inefficient, and slow to change in response to industry trends. The neoprogressive belief in the "scientific management" of health policy was dashed amid protracted conflicts over closing "surplus" hospital beds, turf wars among providers to offer profitable new diagnostic and clinical services, and constant challenges to the adequacy of reimbursement under state rate-setting programs. After more than twenty years of embracing regulatory solutions designed to rationalize the delivery of health care, the financing of health care in the 1990s appeared more irrational than ever.

A growing consensus among policymakers in the 1990s suggests a very different role for state health care regulation than in the past. In recent years, new regulations have responded to emerging trends in the marketplace in an effort to protect patients and providers from the worst excesses of competition. Decision-making authority over the allocation of capital and the rate of payment for health care providers, however, has increasingly been delegated to the private sector. For state agencies, this is a welcome change. Rather than being asked to manage the organization, financing, and delivery of health care in accordance with a systemwide plan, state policymakers now face a more limited, and more achievable, set of goals. Recent experience suggests that competition among providers and health insurers has the potential to control costs; the regulatory challenge for state governments in the 1990s is to harness the powers of the market while protecting the quality of patient care and preserving access to health care for the disadvantaged.

CHAPTER NOTES

1. Uwe Reinhardt (1996) suggests that states' focus on controlling inpatient hospital costs is both ineffective and misplaced. In this view, "a policy of single-mindedly emptying hospitals not only does not save any money, [but] it might even add to total national health spending." Hospital costs would appear less troublesome for policymakers, according to Reinhardt's argument, if payers refocused their negotiations with hospitals on compensating institutions for fixed overhead and the incremental costs associated with a patient's stay rather than flat per diem rates.

2. The intensely negative tone of press coverage and growing public concern over the quality of services provided by MCOs, however, was not mirrored in surveys of plan subscribers, who continued to express a high degree of satisfaction with both their personal physicians and the range and availability of plan services. By 1996, attacks on HMOs had become both routine and highly visible, as several television news magazines (e.g., *Dateline*, *Primetime*

Live) ran prominent stories featuring managed care abuses; *Time* magazine's cover story featured a special report on "What your doctor can't tell you." See Schine and Hammonds (1996), Kuttner (1996), and Keigher (1995) for additional examples of casual stories that presented HMOs as the principal threat to the American health care system.

3. As Bonneyman (1996, 310) notes, "TennCare has been likened to perestroika in the former Soviet bloc: It is a reform process that, once initiated, is difficult to reverse. Indeed, . . . the very chaos and dislocations that TennCare has produced confound those who would turn back the clock."

4. The power to certify MCOs for special-needs populations was part of a larger bill aimed at streamlining implementation of the state's Medicaid managed care waiver (AB 11329); the state's delineation of patient and physician rights appeared in a separate consumer protection bill (SB 7553).

5. See, for example, the guidelines on *Resources for the Optimal Care of the Injured Patient* developed by the American College of Surgeons Committee on Trauma, and the American College of Emergency Physicians' policy statement, *Guidelines for Trauma Care Systems*. Both are regularly updated to reflect changes in technology and medical practice.

6. As a case in point, serious deficiencies in Newport Hospital's clinical laboratory came to light soon after the hospital received glowing reaccreditation reports from both the College of American Pathologists and JCAHO. Neither the accrediting organizations nor the hospital went public with the lab's problems, which first became known when the hospital's liability insurer informed the state Health Department in 1993. For a more extended discussion of the difficulties in regulating the quality of health care services, see Hackey and Williams (1996).

7. The precedent for a formal patient advocacy process already exists in the area of welfare rights, where legal aid programs have represented poor clients since the 1960s.

8. In New York, the state provided two distinct subsidies for uncompensated hospital care prior to 1996. A 5.48% surcharge on inpatient payment rates funded regional uncompensated care pools, while a 1% tax on gross hospital revenues provided funds for a statewide pool to assist distressed hospitals with free care and bad debt. Although the Pataki administration's hospital deregulation bill expanded the surcharge on hospital rates to include outpatient services, it proposed to end payments for bad debt over a three-year period, raising new concerns among providers over the adequacy of the pool. Similar concerns exist in Massachusetts, where the state's uncompensated care pool has been capped at $315 million since 1991; in inflation-adjusted terms, the value of state reimbursement for uncompensated care fell by more than 70% from 1987 to 1994. To make matters worse, Blue Cross and Blue Shield of Massachusetts and other MCOs have eliminated the uncompensated care surcharge in recent contract negotiations with participating hospitals (Demkovich 1996a). In Florida, the state's Public Medical Assistance Trust Fund has also aroused providers' ire, for legislators have expanded the range of providers subject to a 1.5% assessment on net operating revenues to include ambulatory surgical centers, clinical laboratories, and imaging centers as well as hospitals. The surcharge on net revenues is viewed as a particularly onerous

burden by providers for two reasons. On the one hand, since the fund is financed by an "assessment" on revenues rather than a "tax," the state's Agency for Health Care Administration has not permitted providers to pass the cost of the uncompensated care surcharge along to patients and third-party payers. In addition, the revenues generated by the assessment are not redistributed to financially ailing institutions serving a disproportionate number of uninsured patients, but are instead used to defray the state's Medicaid costs (Mikos and Silverstein 1996).

Bibliography

Almond, Gabriel. 1988. The Return to the State. *American Political Science Review* 82: 853–75.

Alter, Joanne, and David Holtzman. 1992. How Outcomes Projects are Changing Medicine. *Business and Health* (Special Issue): 16–23.

Altman, Drew, Richard Greene, and Harvey M. Sapolsky. 1981. *Health Planning and Regulation: The Decision-making Process*. Ann Arbor: AUPHA Press.

Anderson, Gerard, Patrick Chaulk, and Elizabeth Fowler. 1993. Maryland: A Regulatory Approach to Health System Reform. *Health Affairs* 12: 40–47.

Anthony, Robert, and Regina Herzlinger. 1980. *Management Control in the Non-profit Sector*. New York: Academic Press.

Arnold, R. Douglas. 1990. *The Logic of Congressional Action*. New Haven: Yale University Press.

Banham, Russ. 1992. States Are Developing Better Outcomes Data. *Business and Health* (Special Report): 26–28.

Barrow, Clyde W. 1993a. State Autonomy, State Strength, and State Capacities: A Problem of Theory in the New Institutionalism. Paper presented at the annual meeting of the Western Political Science Association held at Pasadena, CA, March 18–20, 1993.

———. 1993b. *Critical Theories of the State*. Madison, WI: University of Wisconsin Press.

Bauder, David. 1992. State Says Private Hospitals Fared Better in '91. *Albany Times-Union* (December 1): B2.

Baumgartner, Frank R., and Bryan D. Jones. 1991. Agenda Dynamics and Policy Subsystems. *Journal of Politics* 53: 1044–1074.

Beauchamp, Dan E. 1993. Waiting for the Big One: Confessions of a Policy Surfer Looking for the Universal Health Care Wave. *Journal of Health Politics, Policy and Law* 18 (1): 203–28.

Beauchamp, Dan E., and Ronald L. Rouse. 1990. Universal New York Health Care. *New England Journal of Medicine* 323: 640–44.

Bentkover, Judith D., Richard E. Schroeder, and A. James Lee. 1985. Effects of Rate Review on the Financial Viability of New York Hospitals: A Retrospective Assessment. Hospital and Health Services Administration 30 (May/June): 94–105.

Berg, John C. 1993. Massachusetts: Citizen Power and Corporate Power. In *Interest Group Politics in the Northeastern States*, Ronald J. Hrebenar and Clive S. Thomas, eds. University Park, PA: Pennsylvania State University Press.

Bergthold, Linda A. 1990a. The Frayed Alliance: Business and Health Care in Massachusetts. *Journal of Health Politics, Policy and Law* 15: 915–18.

———. 1990b. *Purchasing Power in Health: Business, the State and Health Care Politics.* New Brunswick, NJ: Rutgers University Press.

———. 1988. Purchasing Power: Business and Health Policy Change in Massachusetts. *Journal of Health Politics, Policy and Law* 13: 425–51.

Berliner, Howard S., and Sonia Delgado. 1991. The Rise and Fall of New Jersey's Uncompensated Care Fund. *Journal of American Health Policy* 1 (September/October): 47–50.

Bernstein, Marver A. 1955. *Regulating Business Through Independent Commission.* Princeton, NJ: Princeton University Press.

Berry, Jeffrey M. 1994. The Dynamic Qualities of Issue Networks. Paper presented at the 1994 annual meeting of the American Political Science Association in New York, NY, September 1–4.

Beyle, Thad. 1996. Being Governor. In *The State of the States*, 3rd ed., Carl Van Horn, ed. Washington, DC: CQ Press.

———. 1990. Governors. In *Politics in the American States*, 5th ed., Virginia Gray, Herbert Jacob, and Robert Albritton, eds. Glenview, IL: Scott, Foresman/Little Brown.

Biles, B., Carl Schramm, and J. G. Atkinson. 1980. Hospital Cost Inflation Under State Rate-Setting Programs. *New England Journal of Medicine* 303: 664–68.

Bodenheimer, Thomas. 1996. The HMO Backlash: Righteous or Reactionary? *New England Journal of Medicine* 335 (21): 1601–4.

Bonneyman, Gordon. 1996. Stealth Reform: Market-Based Medicaid in Tennessee. *Health Affairs* 15 (2): 306–314.

Boston Globe. 1995. GOP Governors Ask US to Lift Medicaid Rules. *Boston Globe.* June 9: 18.

———. 1991. Putting Hospitals in Jeopardy. *Boston Globe,* November 20: 14.

Bovbjerg, Randall R. 1988. New Directions for Health Planning. In *Cost, Quality, and Access in Health Care*, eds. F. Sloan, J. Blumstein, and J. Perrin, pp. 206–34.

Brace, Paul. 1995. *State Government and Economic Performance.* Baltimore: Johns Hopkins University Press.

Brand, Donald R. 1988. *Corporatism and the Rule of Law.* Ithaca, NY: Cornell University Press.

Brandon, William P. 1991. The Crisis in Health Care Finance in New Jersey. Paper Presented at the Annual Meeting of the American Political Science Association, Washington, DC, 28 August–1 September.

Brecher, Charles. 1984. Medicaid Comes to Arizona: A First Year Report on AHCCCS. *Journal of Health Politics, Policy and Law* 9 (3): 427–52.

Britton, Sharon. 1992. Hospitals Applaud Deregulation Law. *Boston Globe* (January 12): NW1, 6.

Brosco Commission (Rhode Island Commission to Investigate Hospital Room Rates). 1967. *Hospital Costs in Rhode Island: A Report to the Legislature.* Providence, RI: General Assembly.

Brown, David. 1996a. Deluged by Medicaid, States Open Wider Umbrellas. *Washington Post* (June 9): A1.

———. 1996b. When Specialists Aren't the Norm. *Washington Post* (June 10): A1.

———. 1996c. Turning Away Patients as a Way to Survive. *Washington Post* (June 11): A1.

Brown, Lawrence D. 1993. Commissions, Clubs, and Consensus: Reform in Florida. *Health Affairs* 12 (2): 7–26.

———. 1991. Capture and Culture: Organizational Identity in New York Blue Cross. *Journal of Health Politics, Policy and Law* 16 (4): 651–70.

———. 1986. *Health Policy in Transition.* Durham, NC: Duke University Press.

———. 1983. *New Policies, New Politics: Government's Response to Government's Growth.* Washington, DC: Brookings.

———. 1982. Common Sense Meets Implementation: Certificate of Need Regulation in the States. *Journal of Health Politics, Policy and Law* 8: 480–94.

———. 1981. *The Political Structure of the Federal Health Planning Program.* Washington, DC: Brookings.

Brown, Lawrence D., and Catherine McLaughlin. 1990. Constraining Costs at the Community Level. *Health Affairs* 9: 5–28.

Brudney, Jeffrey L., and F. Ted Hebert. 1987. State Agencies and their Environments: Examining the Influence of Important External Actors. *Journal of Politics* 49: 186–206.

Burda, David. 1991. CONspiracies to crush competition. *Modern Healthcare* (July 8): 28–29.

Business Council of New York State. 1996a. February Newsletter (Health Committee). Albany, NY: Author.

———. 1996b. Health Committee Briefing Paper: Health Care Reform. Albany, NY: Author.

———. 1987. Paying the Hospital Bill: Post 1987 Hospital Reimbursement in New York State. Unpublished Manuscript.

Campbell, Ellen S., and Gary M. Fournier. 1993. Certificate-of-Need Deregulation and Indigent Hospital Care. *Journal of Health Politics, Policy and Law* 18: 905–26.

Cannelos, Peter S. 1995. State to Cut Funding for Free Care. *Boston Globe* (December 11): 11.

———. 1991. Panel Modifies Weld Hospital Plan. *Boston Globe* (November 17): 29, 33.

Cantor, Joel C. 1993. Health Care Unreform: The New Jersey Approach. *JAMA* 270 (24): 2968–70.

Cawson, Alan. 1986. *Corporatism and Political Theory.* New York: Basil Blackwell.

Cerne, Frank. 1993. New Hampshire: Hospitals, Physicians, Businesses Converge to Restructure Health Care. *Hospitals and Health Networks* (July 20): 50–51.

Chassin, Marc R., et al. 1987a. Does Inappropriate Use Explain Geographic Variations in the Use of Health Care Services? A Study of Three Procedures. *JAMA* 258 (18): 2533–37.

Chassin, Marc R., et al. 1987b. How Coronary Angiography Is Used: Clinical Determinants of Appropriateness. *JAMA* 258 (18): 2543–47.

232 Bibliography

Chirba-Martin, Mary Ann, and Troyen A. Brennan. 1994. The Critical Role of ERISA in State Health Reform. *Health Affairs* 13 (Spring II): 142–56.
Cingranelli, David L. 1993. New York: Powerful Groups and Powerful Parties. In *Interest Group Politics in the Northeastern States*, Ronald J. Hrebenar and Clive S. Thomas, eds. University Park, PA: Pennsylvania State University Press.
Cleverly, William O. 1993. *The 1993 Almanac of Hospital Financial and Operating Indicators.* Columbus, OH: Center for Healthcare Industry Performance Studies.
Cobb, Roger, and Charles Elder. 1982. *Participation in American Politics*, 2nd ed. Baltimore: Johns Hopkins University Press.
Coelen, Craig G., Gary Gaumer, Philip Burstein, Jerry Cromwell, David Kidder, James Kanak, Nancy Kelly, Ralph Berry, Stephen Mennemeyer, and Eugene Poggio. 1988. *National Hospital Rate Setting Study: Final Report.* Cambridge, MA: Abt Associates.
Colby, Peter W., and John K. White. 1989. Public Policy in New York State Today. In *New York State Today*, Peter Colby and John K. White, eds. Albany, NY: SUNY Press.
Commonwealth of Massachusetts. 1994. *MassHealth: A Request to the Federal Health Care Financing Administration for a Research and Development Waiver Under Section 1115 of the Social Security Act.* Boston: Division of Medical Assistance.
Cornwell, Elmer. 1992. Rhode Island: Bruce Sundlun and the State's Crises. In *Governors and Hard Times*, Thad Beyle, ed., pp. 163–77. Washington, DC: CQ Press.
Cornwell, Elmer, and Maureen Moakley. 1996. The Rhode Island Legislature: An Institution in Transition. Unpublished Manuscript.
Coughlin, Teresa A., Leighton Ku, John Holahan, David Heslam, and Colin Winterbottom. 1994. State Responses to the Medicaid Spending Crisis: 1988 to 1992. *Journal of Health Politics, Policy and Law* 19 (4): 837–64.
Council of State Governments. 1994. *The Book of the States.* Lexington, KY: Council of State Governments.
Couture, Alain. 1988. Analysis of Blue Cross Payments, Medicare Contractual Allowances, and Cost Shift to Blue Cross. Unpublished Table. Concord, NH: Blue Cross and Blue Shield of New Hampshire.
Dana, Maureen McTague. 1986. State Keeping an Eye on Pre-Paid Health Care. *Albany Times-Union* (October 11): 3A.
Dao, James. 1996a. Deadlines Add Tension to Budget Talks. *New York Times* (July 1).
———. 1996b. Albany Accord on Hospitals Propels Budget Talks. *New York Times* (July 1).
———. 1996c. Legislature Finally Ends Its Long Session and Passes Budget. *New York Times* (July 14).
Demkovich, Linda. 1996a. Hospitals Raise Red Flags in the Charity Care Debate. *State Health Notes* 17, No. 228 (May 13): 1–3.
———. 1996b. DeBuono: Leveling the Playing Field. *State Health Notes* 17, No. 228 (May 13): 4.

———. 1996c. Reform Revisited: States Realize Access, Cost Goals. *State Health Notes* 17, No. 234 (August 5): 1–23.

———. 1996d. Hospitals: Full Disclosure? *State Health Notes* 17, No. 232 (July 8): 1–2.

———. 1996e. The Blues: A New Look? *State Health Notes* 17, No. 232 (July 8): 1, 3.

———. 1996f. Rhode Island: Ironing Out the Wrinkles. *State Health Notes* 17, No. 236 (September 16): 1–2.

———. 1995a.Urban Hospitals Face Uncertain Fiscal Times. *State Health Notes* 16, No. 205 (May 29): 1–2.

———. 1995b. Rite Care: Finding Folks "A Medical Home." *State Health Notes* 16, No. 216 (November 13): 1–2.

———. 1994a. Breakthrough or Blackmail? Emotions on TennCare Run High. *State Health Notes* 15, No. 179 (May 2): 1–2, 8.

———. 1994b. Minnesota: Tying Up Loose Ends. *State Health Notes* 15, No. 182 (June 13): 1, 8.

———. 1994c. Vermont: Hitting the Wall. *State Health Notes* 15, No. 182 (June 13): 1–2.

Denn, James. 1996. Health Care on a New Course. *Albany Times-Union* (September 15): C1.

———. 1995. Medicaid Growth Huge in State. *Albany Times-Union* (December 24): B1.

———. 1994. Study Says Private, Non-Profit Hospitals Rebound. *Albany Times-Union* (December 10): B8.

———. 1993. Hospital Losses Growing Despite Healthy Revenues. *Albany Times-Union* (September 19): B1.

Derthick, Martha, and Paul J. Quirk. 1985. *The Politics of Deregulation.* Washington, DC: Brookings.

Dileo, Daniel. 1996. Likely Effects of Devolution on the Redistributive Character of Policy Agendas. *Spectrum: The Journal of State Government* 67 (Summer): 6–15.

Doig, Jameson W., and Erwin C. Hargrove. 1987. *Leadership and Innovation: A Biographical Perspective on Entrepreneurs in Government.* Baltimore: Johns Hopkins University Press.

Donahue, John X., Donald C. Williams, William J. Waters, and Barbara A. DeBuono. 1992. Affordability Considerations in Certificate of Need Hospital Capital Expenditure Review Determinations. *Rhode Island Medicine* 75: 347–50.

Dranove, David. 1993. The Case for Competitive Reform in Health Care. In Richard J. Arnold, Robert Rich, and William White, eds., *Competitive Approaches to Health Care Reform*, pp. 67–82. Washington, DC: Urban Institute Press.

Dunham, Andrew. 1981. Health Regulation: Small Successes, Predictable Failures. Paper presented to the CHAS Health Services Workshop, Feburary 5, 1981.

Dunham, Andrew, and James A. Morone. 1983. *The Politics of Innovation: The Evolution of DRG Rate Regulation in New Jersey.* Princeton, NJ: Health Research and Educational Trust of New Jersey.

Dye, Thomas R. 1984. Party and Policy in the States. *Journal of Politics* 46: 1097–1115.

———. 1966. *Politics, Economics, and the Public: Policy Outcomes in the American States.* Chicago: Rand-McNally.

Easton, David. 1975. A reassessment of the concept of political support. *British Journal of Political Science* 5: 435–57.

Eby, Charles, and D. Cohodes. 1985. What Do We Know About Rate-Setting? *Journal of Health Politics, Policy and Law* 10: 299–327.

Edelman, Lawrence. 1990. Systems Failure. *Boston Globe* (August 21): 21, 27.

Egbert, Robert, and Michelle Anne Fistek. 1993. New Hampshire: Tradition and the Challenge of Growth. In *Interest Group Politics in the Northeastern States,* Ronald J. Hrebenar and Clive S. Thomas, eds. University Park, PA: Pennsylvania State University Press.

Eisner, Marc A. 1993. *Regulatory Politics in Transition.* Baltimore: Johns Hopkins University Press.

Elazar, Daniel. 1974. *American Federalism: A View From the States.* New York: Harper and Row.

Elder, Shirley. 1991. Anger, Frustration Sparked by Hike in Health Insurance Costs. *Boston Globe* (May 19): NH1, 10.

Ellis, Richard J. 1992. Pluralist Political Science and the State: Distinguishing Between Autonomy and Coherence. *Polity* 24: 569–90.

Enthoven, Alain C., and Richard Kronick. 1989a. A Consumer-Choice Health Plan for the 1990s (Part 1). *New England Journal of Medicine* 320 (1): 29–37.

———. 1989b. A Consumer-Choice Health Plan for the 1990s (Part 2). *New England Journal of Medicine* 320: 94–101.

Enthoven, Alain C., and Sarah J. Singer. 1995. Market-Based Reform: What to Regulate and by Whom. *Health Affairs* 14 (Spring): 105–119.

Erikson, Robert S., Gerald Wright, and John C. McIver. 1989. Political Parties, Public Opinion, and State Policy in the United States. *American Political Science Review* 83: 729–50.

Esposito, Alfonso, Michael Hupfer, Cynthia Mason, and Diane Rogler. 1982. Abstracts of State Legislated Hospital Cost-Containment Programs. *Health Care Financing Review* 4 (December): 129–58.

Fiorina, Morris. 1990. *Congress: Keystone of the Washington Establishment,* 2nd ed. New Haven: Yale University Press.

Fishman, Robert M. 1990. Rethinking State and Regime: Southern Europe's Transition to Democracy. *World Politics* 42 (April): 422–442.

Foreman, Howard P., and Bruce L. McClennan. 1996. The Meeting of Managerial Science with Medicine. *JAMA* 276 (19): 1599–1600.

Foster, Richard W. 1982. Cost-Based Reimbursement and Prospective Payment: Reassessing the Incentives. *Journal of Health Politics, Policy and Law* 7: 407–19.

Fowler, Linda, and Robert D. McClure. 1989. *Political Ambition: Who Decides to Run for Congress.* New Haven: Yale University Press.

Fox, Daniel M. 1991. Sharing Governmental Authority: Blue Cross and Hospital Planning in New York City. *Journal of Health Politics, Policy and Law* 16 (4): 719–46.

Fraser, Irene. 1995. Rate Regulation as a Policy Tool: Lessons from New York State. *Health Care Financing Review* 16(3): 151–75.

Freyer, Felice J. 1996. Former Critics Find Much to Praise in R.I.'s Health Care Experiment for the Poor. *Providence Journal-Bulletin* (May 29): 1, 8–9.

———. 1993. Politics Seen Affecting Health Council. *Providence Journal-Bulletin* (October 26): A5.

Friedman, Milton, and Rose Freidman. 1980. *Free to Choose.* New York: Bantam.

Gilbert, Jess, and Carolyn Howe. 1991. Beyond "State vs. Society": Theories of the State and New Deal Agricultural Policies. *American Sociological Review* 56: 204–220.

Ginsberg, Paul B., and Jeremy D. Pickreign. 1996. Tracking Health Care Costs. *Health Affairs* 15 (3): 140–49.

Gold, Steven. 1994. *The Fiscal Crisis of the States.* Washington, DC: Georgetown University Press.

Goldberg, Lawrence G., and Warren Greenberg. 1995. The Response of the Dominant Firm to Competition: The Ocean State Case. *Health Care Management Review* 20 (1): 65–74.

Goldberger, Susan A. 1990. The Politics of Universal Access: The Massachusetts Health Security Act of 1988. *Journal of Health Politics, Policy and Law* 15: 857–86.

Gormley, William T. 1986. Regulatory Issue Networks in a Federal System. *Polity* 18: 595–620.

Gostin, Lawrence O. 1996. Law and Medicine. *JAMA* 275 (23): 1817–19.

Gottlieb, Martin. 1993. Enrollment Diminishes at Blue Cross. *New York Times* (September 4): 21.

Gray, Virginia, and David Lowery. 1993. The Diversity of State Interest Group Systems. *Political Research Quarterly* 46: 81–97.

———. 1991. Corporatism Without Labor? Industrial Policy Making in the American States. *Journal of Public Policy* 11: 315–329.

———. 1990. The Corporatist Foundations of State Industrial Policy. *Social Science Quarterly* 71: 3–23.

Grayboys, Thomas B., Beth Biegelsen, Steven Lampert, Charles Blatt, and Bernard Lown. 1992. Results of a Second-Opinion Trial Among Patients Recommended for Coronary Angiography. *JAMA* 268: 2537–2540.

Grogan, Colleen. 1995. Hope in Federalism? What Can the States Do and What Are They Likely to Do? *Journal of Health Politics, Policy and Law* 20(2): 477–85.

Grunwald, Michael. 1996. Quietly, Weld Aides Rewrite the State's Rulebook. *Boston Globe* (October 3): A1, A14–15.

Gustis, Philip S. 1989. What Might Be Done to Cut Losses for New York's Hospitals. *New York Times* (June 25): E5.

Guterman, Stuart, Jack Ashby, and Timothy Greene. 1996. Hospital Cost Growth Down. *Health Affairs* 15 (3): 134–39.

Hacker, Jacob S. 1996. National Health Care Reform: An Idea Whose Time Came and Went. *Journal of Health Politics, Policy and Law* 21 (4): 647–96.

Hackey, Robert B. 1993a. The Illogic of Health Care Reform: Policy Dilemmas for the 1990s. *Polity* 26 (Winter): 233–58.

———. 1993b. New Wine in Old Bottles: Certificate of Need in the 1990s. *Journal of Health Politics, Policy and Law* 18 (Winter): 927–36.

———. 1993c. Regulatory Regimes and State Rate Setting Programs. *Journal of Health Politics, Policy and Law* 18 (Summer): 491–502.

———. 1992. Trapped Between State and Market: Regulating Hospital Payment in the Northeastern States. *Medical Care Review* 49 (Fall): 355–88.

Hackey, Robert B., and Peter F. Fuller. 1995. Life After Death: Certificate-of-Need Revisited. Unpublished Manuscript.

Hackey, Robert B., and Donald C. Williams. 1996. Hard Choices in Health Care Regulation: Monitoring the Quality of Hospital Laboratory Services. In *Ethical Dilemmas in Public Administration*, Lynn Pasquerella, Alfred G. Killilea, and Michael Vocino, eds. Westport, CT: Greenwood Press.

Hadley, Jack. 1988. Medicare Spending and Mortality Rates of the Elderly. *Inquiry* 25: 485–93.

Hadley, Jack, and Kathy Swartz. 1989. The Impact on Hospital Costs Between 1980 and 1984 of Hospital Rate Regulation, Competition, and Changes in Health Insurance Coverage. *Inquiry* 26: 35–47.

Hale, Dennis. 1992. Massachusetts: William F. Weld and the End of Business as Usual. In Thad Beyle, ed., *Governors and Hard Times*. Washington, DC: CQ Press.

Hanafin, Teresa. 1991a. Full House OK's Health Care Finance Bill. *Boston Globe* (November 20): 88.

———. 1991b. Massachusetts House Rejects Single-Payer Insurance. *Boston Globe* (November 21): 82.

———. 1991c. Hospital Finance Bill Decried as Capitulation to Weld. *Boston Globe* (September 19): 49.

Hanson, Russell L. 1994. Health Care Reform, Managed Competition, and Subnational Politics. *Publius: The Journal of Federalism* 24 (Summer): 49–69.

Harris, Norma. 1994a. Are Health Plans Making the Grade? *Business and Health* (June): 22–28.

———. 1994b. How Hospitals Measure Up. *Business and Health* (August): 20–24.

Harris, Richard, and Sidney Milikis. 1989. *The Politics of Regulatory Change*. New York: Oxford University Press.

Harrop, Froma. 1996. Yankee GOPers Go Democratic. *Providence Journal-Bulletin* (November 26): B7.

Healthcare Association of New York State. 1996. Proposed 1996–97 NYS Budget: Implications for Providers and Consumers. Albany, NY: Author.

———. 1995. New York State Legislative Summary. Albany, NY: Author.

Health Care Financing Administration (HCFA). 1996a. Massachusetts Statewide Health Reform Demonstration Fact Sheet. Washington, DC: HCFA.

———. 1996c. New Hampshire Statewide Health Reform Demonstration Fact Sheet (Revised July 5, 1996). Washington, DC: HCFA.

———. 1996d. Rhode Island Statewide Health Reform Demonstration Fact Sheet. Washington, DC: HCFA.

———. 1988. *Medicare and Medicaid Data Book, 1988*. Washington, DC: U.S. Government Printing Office.

Heclo, Hugh. 1978. Issue Networks and the Executive Establishment. In Anthony King, ed., *The New American Political System*, pp. 87–124. Washington, DC: American Enterprise Institute.

———. 1974. *Modern Social Politics in Britain and Sweden*. New Haven: Yale University Press.

Hellinger, Fred J. 1996. The Expanding Scope of State Legislation. *JAMA* 276 (13): 1065–70.

———. 1985. Recent Evidence on Case-Based Systems for Setting Hospital Rates. *Inquiry* 22 (Spring): 78–91.

———. 1976. Prospective Reimbursement through Budget Review: New Jersey, Rhode Island, and Western Pennsylvania. *Inquiry* 13: 309–20.

Herman, Robin. 1981. Governor Calls Medicaid First Legislative Priority. *New York Times* (May 27): B2.

Hernandez, Raymond. 1996. Frustrated N.Y. Legislators Know When to Vote, Not for What. *New York Times* (July 2).

Hevesi, Alan G. 1989. The Renewed Legislature. In *New York State Today*, Peter Colby and John K. White, eds. Albany, NY: SUNY Press.

———. 1975. *Legislative Politics in New York State: A Comparative Analysis*. New York: Praeger.

Higgs, Robert. 1987. *Crisis and Leviathan: Critical Episodes in the Growth of American Government*. New York: Oxford University Press.

Hilborne, Lee H., Lucian Leape, Steven Bernstein, Rolla Edward Park, Mary Fiske, Caren J. Kamberg, Carol Pinder Roth, and Robert H. Brook. 1993. The Appropriateness of Use of Percutaneous Tranluminal Coronary Angioplasty in New York State. *JAMA* 269 (6): 761–65.

Holbrook-Provow, Thomas M., and Steven C. Poe. 1987. Measuring State Political Ideology. *American Politics Quarterly* 15: 399–416.

Hooks, Gregory. 1990. From an Autonomous to a Captured State Agency: The Decline of the New Deal in Agriculture. *American Sociological Review* 55: 29–43.

Hospital Association of New York State. 1990a. Hospital Reimbursement in New York State: A Historical Perspective. Unpublished Working Paper. Albany, NY: Author.

———. 1990b. *Regulatory Reform: Towards a More Effective Health Care System*. Albany, NY: Author.

Hospital Association of Rhode Island. 1986. Obligations of Hospitals to Negotiate Budgets. Advisory memorandum to William Sweeney from Hinckley, Allen, Tobin and Silverstein.

Howe, Peter J. 1991. Weld Hones Axe for Rules Seen as Impeding Firms. *Boston Globe* (September 21): 36.

Howitt, Arnold M., and R. Clifford Leftwich. 1987. Massachusetts. In *Reagan and the States*, Richard P. Nathan and Fred C. Doolittle, eds. Princeton, NJ: Princeton University Press.

Hudson, William, Mark Hyde, and John Carroll. 1992. The Entrepreneurial State Goes to Europe: State Economic Policies and Europe 1992. *New England Journal of Public Policy* 9 (1): 19–32.

Humbert, Marc. 1992. Cuomo Hints at State Pay Hike. *Albany Times-Union* (January 15): A1.

Huntington, Samuel. 1968. *Political Order in Changing Societies*. New Haven: Yale University Press.

Hyde, Mark. 1993. Rhode Island: The Politics of Intimacy. In *Interest Group Politics in the Northeastern States*, Ronald J. Hrebenar and Clive S. Thomas, eds. University Park, PA: Pennsylvania State University Press.

Ikenberry, G. John. 1988. *Reasons of State: Oil Politics and the Capacities of American Government*. Ithaca, NY: Cornell University Press.

Imershein, Allen W., Philip C. Rond III, and Mary P. Mathis. 1992. Restructuring Patterns of Elite Dominance and the Formation of State Policy in Health Care. *American Journal of Sociology* 97 (4): 970–93.

Intergovernmental Health Policy Project. 1994. *State Profiles: Health Care Reform*, 2nd ed. (February). Washington, DC: The George Washington University.

Jacobs, Lawrence. 1992. Institutions and Culture: Health Policy and Public Opinion in the U.S. and Britain. *World Politics* 44: 179–209.

Jacobs, Sally. 1996. Jeanne Shaheen's Journey. *Boston Globe* (November 14), A1, A20-A21.

Jensen, Dorothy A., Amanda H. McCloskey, and Rolando Fuentes. 1994. *Reforming the Health Care System: State Profiles 1994*. Washington, DC: American Association of Retired Persons Public Policy Institute.

Jewell, Malcolm. 1982. The Neglected World of State Politics. *Journal of Politics* 44: 638–57.

Jimenez, Ralph. 1994. Hospitals Turn to Liens to Collect Fees. *Boston Globe* (February 27): NH1, 9.

———. 1993. State First, Last on Medicaid. *Boston Globe* (January 31) NH1, 6.

———. 1992a. Some Hospitals May Be Skirting Rule on Windfall from Medicaid. *Boston Globe* (April 5): NH1, 17.

———. 1992b. Hospitals United on Planned Clinic. *Boston Globe* (April 5): NH17.

———. 1991. Hospital Bows to Welfare Group. *Boston Globe* (May 12): NH1, 14.

———. 1990. Insurers Seek a Cure in State for a Dilemma. *Boston Globe* (December 8): NH1, 8.

Jones, Brian C. 1996. Debate Over Hospitals to Heat Up. *Providence Journal-Bulletin* (December 29): A1, 14.

Jones, Charles O. 1968. The Minority Party and Policy-making in the House of Representatives. *American Political Science Review* 62: 481–93.

Jones, Rich. 1995. State Legislatures. *Book of the States* (1994–95): 98–107.

Jordan, Karen A. 1996. Travelers Insurance: New Support for the Argument to Restrain ERISA Pre-emption. *Yale Journal on Regulation* 13 (1): 255–336.

Joskow, Paul L. 1981. *Controlling Hospital Costs: The Role of Government Regulation*. Cambridge, MA: MIT Press.

Kaiser Commision on the Future of Medicaid. 1995. *Medicaid Special Financing Arrangements: Disproportionate Share Hospital (DSH) Payments, Provider Taxes, and Intergovernmental Transfers*. Washington, DC: Author.

Karlin, Rick. 1993. Health Chief Focuses on "Quality Measurement." *Albany Times-Union* (March 8): B2.

Keigher, Sharon M. 1995. Managed Care's Silent Seduction of America and the New Politics of Choice. *Health and Social Work* 20 (2): 146–51.

Kiernan, Laura A. 1991. Health Care: Grim Gets Grimmer. *Boston Globe* (June 30): NH1, 10.

Kinney, Eleanor D. 1987. Coordinating Rate Setting and Planning in States with Mandatory Hospital Rate Regulation: What Makes a Difference? *Journal of Legal Medicine* 8: 397–435.

Kirkman-Liff, Bradford L. 1991. Health Insurance Values and Implementation in the Netherlands and the Federal Republic of Germany. *JAMA* 265: 2496–2502.

Klingman, David, and William Lammers. 1984. The "General Policy Liberalism" Factor in American State Politics. *American Journal of Political Science* 28: 598–610.

Knox, Richard A. 1996a. Health Coverage Debated on Hill. *Boston Globe* (January 17): 19.

———. 1996b. Blue Cross Gives Jolt to Hospitals. *Boston Globe* (January 29): 1, 22.

———. 1994a. AG Pushes Hospitals on Charity Services. *Boston Globe* (January 25): 17, 19.

———. 1994. More Oversight Over Hospital Mergers Urged. *Boston Globe* (November 22): 41.

———. 1993b. Hospitals' Riches: Excess or Necessity? *Boston Globe* (May 9): 1, 10.

———. 1991a. Let Hospitals Compete, Weld Says. *Boston Globe* (July 4): 14.

———. 1991b. Weld Plan to Deregulate Hospitals Decried. *Boston Globe* (October 4): 22.

———. 1991c. Democrats Follow Weld on Hospital Bill. *Boston Globe* (September 22): 25–26.

———. 1991d. Dueling Memos Heighten Battle Over Mass. Hospital Deregulation. *Boston Globe* (November 20): 88.

———. 1991e. Harvard's Nancy Kane Says Hospitals are Profit Poor But Cash Rich. *Boston Globe* (February 3): 73, 75.

———. 1990a. Hospital Industry Rejects Deregulation. *Boston Globe* (December 5): 1, 24.

———. 1989a. Neglect Threatens Health Law, Panel Says. *Boston Globe* (April 11): 23.

———. 1988. Universal Health Care Bill Passes. *Boston Globe* (April 14): 1.

———. 1987a. Employer Tax Sought for Health Insurance. *Boston Globe* (August 6): 1, 10.

———. 1987b. A Dilemma for the State's Hospitals. *Boston Globe* (October 5): 1, 9.

———. 1987c. Study: Hospitals Seeing Profits. *Boston Globe* (May 22): 23, 29.

———. 1987d. Health Bill Advances. *Boston Globe* (October 1): 25, 30.

Kolbert, Elizabeth. 1991. New York Medicaid Costs Surge, But Health Care for the Poor Lags. *New York Times* (April 14): 1, 26.

———. 1988. New York Extending Medicaid Eligibility and Shifting Services. *New York Times* (August 25): B1.

Kolko, Gabriel. 1965. *Railroads and Regulation: 1877–1916*. New York: Norton.

Kong, Dolores. 1995. Beacon Hill Reopens Health Care Debate. *Boston Globe* (May 1): 17, 20.

———. 1991. Managed Care: Solution or Euphemism? *Boston Globe* (July 15): 25.

Kong, Dolores, and Gerard O'Neill. 1996. State Will Tell New For-Profit Hospitals to Keep Free Care. *Boston Globe* (November 20): A1, A21.

KPMG Peat Marwick LLP. 1996. *The Impact of Managed Care on U.S. Markets: Executive Summary*. New York: KPMG Peat Marwick.

Krasner, Stephen D. 1983. Structural Causes and Regime Consequences: Regimes as Intervening Variables. In *International Regimes*, Stephen Krasner, ed. Ithaca, NY: Cornell University Press.

———. 1978. *Defending the National Interest*. Princeton, NJ: Princeton University Press.

Kronick, Richard. 1992. Commentary: Can Consumer Choice Reward Quality and Economy? Towards a Test of Economic Competition. *Journal of Health Politics, Policy and Law* 17: 25–34.

———. 1990. The Slippery Slope of Health Care Finance: Business Interests and Hospital Reimbursement in Massachusetts. *Journal of Health Politics, Policy and Law* 15: 887–914.

Ku, Leighton, and Teresa A. Coughlin. 1994. *Medicaid Disproportionate Share and Other Special Financing Programs: A Fiscal Dilemma for States and the Federal Government*. Washington, DC: Kaiser Commission on the Future of Medicaid.

Kuttner, Robert. 1996. Who Manages the Managers? *Boston Globe* (November 25): 15.

Langley, Monica, and Anita Sharpe. 1996. IRS, State Officials, and Courts Get Involved, Tangling Deals. *Wall Street Journal Interactive Edition* (October 18): Online.

Lawson, Stephanie. 1993. Conceptual Issues in the Comparative Study of Regime Change and Democratization. *Comparative Politics*: 183–205.

Leape, Lucian L., Lee H. Hilborne, Rolla Edward Park, Steven Bernstein, Caren J. Kamberg, Marjorie Sherwood, and Robert H. Brook. 1993. The Appropriateness of Use of Coronary Artery Bypass Graft Surgery in New York State. *JAMA* 269 (6): 753–60.

Leco, Armand P. 1976. Prospective Rate Setting in Rhode Island. *Topics in Health Care Financing* 3 (2): 39–56.

Leichter, Howard M. 1993a. Health Care Reform in Vermont: A Work in Progress. *Health Affairs* 12 (2): 71–81.

———. 1993b. Minnesota: The Trip from Acrimony to Accommodation. *Health Affairs* 12 (2): 48–58.

Letsch, Suzanne W. 1993. National Health Care Spending in 1991. *Health Affairs* 12 (1): 94–110.

Levit, Katharine R., Helen C. Lazenby, and Lekha Sivarajan. 1996. Health Care Spending in 1994: Slowest in Decades. *Health Affairs* 15 (2): 130–44.

Levit, Katharine R., et al. 1993. Health Spending by State: New Estimates for Policy Making. *Health Affairs* 12 (3): 7–20.

Lewin, Lawrence S., Anne R. Somers, and Herman M. Somers. 1975. State Health Cost Regulation: Structure and Administration. *University of Toledo Law Review* 6: 647–76.

Liebschutz, Sarah F., and Irene Lurie. 1987. New York. In *Reagan and the States*, pp. 169–207, Richard P. Nathan and Fred C. Doolittle, eds. Princeton, NJ: Princeton University Press.

Lindberg, Gregory et al. 1988. Health Care Cost Containment Measures and Mortality in Hennepin County's Medicaid Elderly and All Elderly. *American Journal of Public Health* 79: 1481–85.

Lipman, Harvey. 1996a. Hospitals Face $1B in Medicaid Reductions. *Albany Times-Union* (June 28): B2.

———. 1996b. Senate Weighs in with Hospital Funding Legislation. *Albany Times-Union* (June 12): B2.

Little, Jane Sneddon. 1991. Medicaid. *New England Economic Review* (January/February): 27–50.

Lochhead, Terry. 1991. The State and Medicare: How Not to Use a Loophole. *Boston Globe* (December 1): NH5.

Lockard, Duane. 1959. *New England State Politics*. Princeton, NJ: Princeton University Press.

Loth, Renee. 1989. Hospitals Sue State Over Medical Bills. *Boston Globe* (August 16): 30.

Lowery, David, and Virginia Gray. 1993. The Density of State Interest Group Systems. *Journal of Politics* 55 (1): 191–206.

Lowery, David, and Lee Sigelman. 1982. Political Culture and State Public Policy: The Missing Link. *Western Political Quarterly* 35: 376–84.

Lowi, Theodore. 1969. *The End of Liberalism*. New York: Norton.

Luft, Harold F., Susan C. Maerki, and Joan B. Trauner. 1986. The Competitive Effects of Health Maintenance Organizations: Another Look at the Evidence from Hawaii, Rochester, and Minneapolis/St. Paul. *Journal of Health Politics, Policy and Law* 10: 625–58.

Lundburg, George. 1992. National Health Care Reform: The Aura of Inevitabilty Intensifies. *JAMA* 267: 2524.

Marion Merrill Dow, Inc. 1994. Managed Care Digest, HMO Edition, 1994. *Medical Benefits* 11 (20): 1–2.

Marmor, Theodore R. 1991. New York's Blue Cross and Blue Shield, 1934–1990: The Complicated Politics of Nonprofit Regulation. *Journal of Health Politics, Policy and Law* 16 (4): 761–92.

Marmor, Theodore, and James A. Morone. 1981. Representing Consumer Interests: The Case of American Health Planning. *Ethics* 91: 431–50.

Marmor, Theodore, Donald Wittman, and Thomas Heagy. 1976. The Politics of Medical Inflation. *Journal of Health Politics, Policy and Law* 1: 69–85.

Martin, Cathie Jo. 1993. Together Again: Business, Government, and the Quest for Cost Control. *Journal of Health Politics, Policy and Law* 18 (2): 359–94.

Mashek, John, and Frank Philips. 1991. Despite US Budget Chief's Dig, Some Medicaid Funds Roll In. *Boston Globe* (June 4): 18.

May, Peter J. 1991. Reconsidering Policy Design: Policies and Publics. *Journal of Public Policy* 11 (2): 187–206.

Mayhew, D. 1974. *Congress: The Electoral Connection*. New Haven: Yale University Press.

McConnell, Grant. 1966. *Private Power and American Democracy*. New York: Vintage.

McDonough, John E. 1995. Tracking the Demise of State Hospital Rate Setting. Unpublished manuscript.

McDonough, John E., Christie Hager, and Brian Rosman. 1997. Health Care Reform Stages a Comeback in Massachusetts. *New England Journal of Medicine* 336 (2): 148–51.

McLaughlin, Catherine G., Wendy Zellers, and Lawrence D. Brown. 1989. Health Care Coalitions: Characteristics, Activities, and Prospects. *Inquiry* 26: 72–83.

McNamara, Eileen. 1996. Public Spirit on Health Front. *Boston Globe* (October 30): B1.

Meier, Barry. 1993. Empire's Problems Suggest Hurdles for Managed Care. *New York Times* (August 23): 17.

Meier, Kenneth J. 1985. *Regulation: Politics, Bureaucracy, and Economics.* New York: St. Martin's.

Mendelson, Daniel N., Richard G. Abramson, and Robert J. Rubin. 1995. States and Technology Assessment. *Health Affairs* 14 (2): 83–98.

Meyer, Gregg S., and David Blumenthal. 1996. TennCare and Academic Medical Centers. *JAMA* 276 (9): 672–76.

Migdal, Joel S. 1988. *Strong Societies and Weak States.* Princeton, NJ: Princeton University Press.

Mikos, Cynthia, and Murray B. Silverstein. 1996. Defects in the Indigent Health Care Trust Fund. *Tampa Bay Business Journal* (August 26). Online.

Milne, John. 1992. Health Care White Papers. *Boston Globe* (August 9): NH1, 6.

———. 1991. Medicaid Rules May Help State to Extra $200m. *Boston Globe* (November 10): NH1, 8.

Mirvis, David M., Cyril F. Chang, Christopher J. Hall, Gregory T. Zaar, and William B. Applegate. 1995. TennCare—Health System Reform for Tennessee. *JAMA* 274 (15): 1235–41.

Mitchell, Samuel A. 1988. Issues, Evidence, and the Policymaker's Dilemma. *Health Affairs* : 84–97.

Mohl, Bruce. 1989a. Budget Battle Moves to Senate. *Boston Globe* (March 16): 1, 38.

Morone, James A. 1992. Hidden Complications: Why Health Care Needs Regulation. *The American Prospect* 10 (Summer): 40–48.

———. 1990. *The Democratic Wish: Representation and Reform in American Politics.* New York: Basic Books.

Morone, James A., and Andrew Dunham. 1985. Slouching Towards National Health Insurance: The New Health Care Politics. *Yale Journal on Regulation* 2: 263–91.

———. 1984. The Waning of Professional Dominance: DRGs and the Hospitals. *Health Affairs* 3: 73–84.

Mueller, Keith J. 1988. Federal Programs to Expire: The Case of Health Planning. *Public Administration Review* 48: 719–25.

Murphy, Shelly. 1996. Weld Counters with Own Health Plan. *Boston Globe* (May 5): 30.

National Committee for Quality Assurance. 1996. *HEDIS 3.0 Executive Summary.* Online at http://www.ncqa.org/hedis/30execsum.htm.

New Hampshire Health Services Planning and Review Board. 1992. *Annual Data Report, November 1992.* Concord, NH: Author.

New Hampshire Hospital Association. 1990. *The Facts: Hospitals in New Hampshire, 1983–1988.* Concord, NH: Author.

New York Conference of Blue Cross and Blue Shield Plans v. Travelers Insurance Company et al. 1995. *Supreme Court Reporter* 115: 1671–83.

New York State. 1995. *The Partnership Plan: A Public-Private Initiative Ensuring Healthcare for Needy New Yorkers.* Albany, NY: Governor's Office.

New York State Department of Health. 1995a. *Coronary Artery Bypass Surgery in New York State, 1991–1993.* Albany, NY: Department of Health.

———. 1995b. *New Directions for a Healthier New York: Reform of the Health Care Financing System.* Albany, NY: Department of Health.

———. 1993. *New York Health.* Unpublished Newsletter. Albany, NY: Department of Health.

———. 1990a. Universal New York Health Care: A Proposal (Revision I). Unpublished Manuscript. Albany, NY: Department of Health.

———. 1990b. The Hospital Case-Based Payment System, 1988–90. Unpublished Manuscript. Albany, NY: Office of Health Systems Management.

Nordlinger, Eric A. 1981. *On the Autonomy of the Democratic State.* Cambridge, MA: Harvard University Press.

Offe, Claus. 1981. The Attribution of Public Status to Interest Groups. In Suzanne Berger, ed., *Organizing Interests in Western Europe,* pp. 123–58. Cambridge: Cambridge University Press.

Pataki, George. 1995. Partisanship a 2-Way Street. *Albany Times-Union* (January 5): A7.

Pauly, Mark V., Patricia Danzon, Paul Feldstein, and John Hoff. 1991. A Plan for "Responsible National Health Insurance." *Health Affairs* 10 (1): 5–25.

Peirce, Neal R. 1976. *The New England States: People, Politics, and Power in the Six New England States.* New York: Norton.

Pennsylvania Health Care Cost Containment Council. 1992. *A Consumer's Guide to Coronary Artery Bypass Graft Surgery.* Harrisburg, PA: Author.

Perkins, Jane. 1985. The Effects of Health Care Cost Containment on the Poor: An Overview. *Clearinghouse Review* 19 (December): 831–52.

Pham, Alex. 1996a. Harvard, Matthew Thornton Seek Merger. *Boston Globe* (December 10): C1, C16.

———. 1996b. Prescribing a Merger. *Boston Globe* (December 6): C1, C5.

———. 1996c. HMOs Facing Unexpected Costs Surge. *Boston Globe* (August 2): A1.

———. 1996d. Blue Cross Pushes for State Help. *Boston Globe* (October 4): C1, C5.

Picchi, Joe. 1994. Hoblock, Buono Demand Action on Medicaid. *Albany Times-Union* (April 5): B4.

Plotnick, Robert D., and Richard F. Winters. 1985. A Politico-Economic Theory of Income Redistribution. *American Political Science Review* 79: 458–73.

Prechel, Harlan. 1990. Conflict and Historical Variation in Steel Capital-State Relations: The Emergence of State Structures and a More Prominent, Less Autonomous State. *American Sociological Review* 55: 693–98.

Precious, Tom. 1992. The Doctor Is In, at $98,399. *Albany Times-Union* (June 10): B8.

Providence Journal-Bulletin. 1996. Wrong Place for a For-Profit (December 15): D14.

Pulliam, Susan. 1991. Blue Cross Beset by Financial Problems. *Wall Street Journal* (March 27): A6.

Read, Charles J. 1996. State No. 1 in Cost Effectiveness. *Providence Business News* (February 12): 1, 17.

Reinhardt, Uwe. 1996. Spending More Through "Cost Control": Our Obsessive Quest to Gut the Hospital. *Health Affairs* 15 (2): 145–53.

Robertson, David Brian. 1993. The Return to History and the New Institutionalism in American Political Science. *Social Science History* 17 (1): 1–36.

Robinson, James C. 1991. HMO Market Penetration and Hospital Cost Inflation in California. *JAMA* 266 (19): 2719–24.

Robinson, James C., and Harold S. Luft. 1988. Competition, Regulation, and Hospital Costs, 1982 to 1986. *JAMA* 260 (18): 2676–81.

Rochefort, David A., and Roger W. Cobb. *The Politics of Problem Definition.* Lawrence, KS: University Press of Kansas.

Rochefort, David A., and Paul J. Pezza. 1992. Public Opinion and Health Care Policy. In *Health Politics and Policy*, 2nd ed., ed. T. J. Litman and L. Robins, pp. 247–70. Albany, NY: Delmar.

Rodwin, Marc A. 1996. Consumer Protection and Managed Care: The Need for Organized Consumers. *Health Affairs* 15 (3): 110–23.

Roemer, Milton I. 1961. Bed Supply and Hospital Utilization: A Natural Experiment. *Hospitals* 35 (November 1): 37.

Roos, Roberta M. 1987. Certificate of Need for Health Care Facilities: A Time for Re-examination. *Pace Law Review* 7: 491–530.

Rosenbaum, Sara, and Julie Darnell. 1995. *Medicaid Section 1115 Demonstration Waivers: Implications for Federal Legislative Reform.* Washington, DC: Kaiser Commission on the Future of Medicaid.

Rosenstone, Steven J. 1983. *Forecasting Presidential Elections.* New Haven: Yale University Press.

Rosenthal, Alan. 1996. The Legislature: Unraveling of Institutional Fabric. In *The State of the States*, 3rd ed., Carl Van Horn, ed. Washington, DC: CQ Press.

Ross, Robert H., and Donna M. Bright. 1996. Documenting the Boston City Hospital and Boston University Medical Center Hospital Merger: A Case Study. Paper presented to the annual meeting of the New England Political Science Association in Springfield, MA.

Rothenberg, Eleanore. 1974. *Regulation and Expansion of Health Facilities: The Certificate of Need Experience in New York State.* New York: Praeger.

Rovner, Julie. 1992. "Pay or Play" Gains Momentum as Labor Panel Marks Up Bill. *Congressional Quarterly Weekly Report* (January 25): 172–74.

Sack, Kevin. 1991. Health Chief's Illness Leaves Albany Policies in Doubt. *New York Times* (April 1): B1, B7.

Sage, William M. 1996. "Health Law 2000": The Legal System and the Changing Health Care Market. *Health Affairs* 15 (3): 9–27.

Sager, Alan. 1988. Prices of Equitable Access: The New Massachusetts Health Insurance Law. *Hastings Center Report* (June/July): 21–25.

Sahlein, William J. 1973. *Prospective Rate Setting for Hospital Care Provided to Publicly Aided Patients.* Unpublished Report: Executive Office for Administration and Finance, Commonwealth of Massachusetts.

Salisbury, Robert H. 1979. Why No Corporatism in America? In Phillipe Schmitter and Gerhard Lembruch, eds., *Trends Towards Corporatist Intermediation*, pp. 212–29. Beverly Hills, CA: Sage.

Salkever, David, and Thomas Bice. 1981. *Hospital Certificate of Need Controls: Impact on Investment, Costs, and Use.* Washington, DC: American Enterprise Institute.

Sanchez, Rosalee. 1996a. Reform Revisited: TennCare Still Stirs Patient, Provider Concerns. *State Health Notes* 17 (No. 235): 1–2.

Sapolsky, Harvey M. 1991a. The Democratic Wish: A Symposium. *Journal of Health Politics, Policy and Law* 16 (4): 821–22.

———. 1991b. Empire and the Business of Health Insurance. *Journal of Health Politics, Policy and Law* 16 (4): 747–60.

———. 1986. Prospective Payment in Perspective. *Journal of Health Politics, Policy and Law* 11 (4): 633–46.

Sapolsky, Harvey M., James Aisenberg, and James A. Morone. 1987. The Call to Rome and Other Obstacles to State Level Innovation. *Public Administration Review*: 135–142.

Schine, Eric, and Keith H. Hammonds. 1996. In California, It's 'Hell No, HMO!' *Business Week* (May 20): 38.

Schmitter, Phillipe C. 1979. "Still the Century of Corporatism?" in *Trends Towards Corporatist Intermediation*, Schmitter and Lembruch, eds. Beverly Hills, CA: Sage Publications.

Schultze, Charles L. 1977. *The Public Use of Private Interest.* Washington, DC: Brookings.

Scott, H. Denman, John T. Tierney, William J. Waters, Donald C. Williams, and John X. Donohue. 1987. Certificate of Need: A State Perspective. *Rhode Island Medical Journal* 70: 341–45.

Sessler, Amy. 1994. Dying Hospitals Find New Leases on Life. *Boston Globe* (February 7): 25, 27.

Skocpol, Theda. 1993. *Protecting Soldiers and Mothers.* Cambridge, MA: Harvard University Press.

———. 1985. Bringing the State Back In: Strategies of Analysis in Current Research. In Peter Evans, Dietrich Rueschmeyer, and Theda Skocpol, eds, *Bringing the State Back In*, pp. 3–37. Cambridge, MA: Cambridge University Press.

Skowronek, Stephen. 1982. *Building a New American State.* New York: Cambridge University Press.

Sloan, Frank A. 1988. Containing Health Expenditures: Lessons Learned from Certificate of Need Programs. In *Cost, Quality, and Access in Health Care*, eds. F. Sloan, J. Blumstein, and J. Perrin, pp. 44–70.

———. 1983. Rate Regulation as a Strategy for Hospital Cost Control: Evidence From the Last Decade. *Milbank Memorial Fund Quarterly/Health and Society* 61: 195–216.

———. 1981. Regulation and the Rising Cost of Hospital Care. *Review of Economics and Statistics* 63: 479–487.

Smith, Paul A. 1984. New York. In *The Political Life of the American States*, Maureen Moakley and Alan Rosenthan, eds., pp. 247–75. New York: Praeger.

Sparer, Michael S. 1996. *Medicaid and the Limits of State Health Care Reform.* Philadelphia: Temple University Press.

Starr, Paul. 1982. *The Social Transformation of American Medicine*. New York: Basic Books.

Starr, Paul, and Walter Zelman. 1993. Bridge to Compromise: Competition Under a Budget. *Health Affairs* 11 (Supplement): 7–23.

State of New Hampshire, Department of Health and Human Services. 1996. *State of New Hampshire Medicaid Demonstration Waiver Application: Community Care Systems*. Concord, NH: Author.

State of Rhode Island. 1993. *RIte Care: A Proposal for the Development of a Statewide Demonstration Project*. Providence, RI: Office of the Governor.

State of Rhode Island, Special Legislative Commission to Study Health Care Capital Expenditures. 1983. *Final Report*. Anthony J. Carceri, Chair. Providence, RI: General Assembly.

Stein, Charles. 1996a. Massachusetts Hospitals Post Gains; Cuts in Costs Cited. *Boston Globe* (February 2): 27.

———. 1996b. Report Says Health Care Safety Net Torn. *Boston Globe* (September 25): E2.

———. 1996c. Top Quality HMOs Not Rated the Most Popular. *Boston Globe* (April 2): 37, 49.

———. 1994. Weld Medicaid Plan Endorsed by Study. *Boston Globe* (June 29): 37.

———. 1993. Tackling the Medicaid Budget Buster. *Boston Globe* (March 21): 77, 94.

———. 1992. The Health Care Bargain Hunt. *Boston Globe* (July 7): 33, 38.

———. 1991a. Massachusetts Hospitals Singing the Blues. *Boston Globe* (October 24): 49–50.

———. 1991b. Pushing Hospitals to Compete. *Boston Globe* (July 14): 29, 33.

———. 1990a. Hospital Group Sues State Over New Debt Rule. *Boston Globe* (June 8): 27, 30.

Steinmo, Sven, and Jon Watts. 1995. It's the Institutions, Stupid! Why Comprehensive National Health Insurance Always Fails in America. *Journal of Health Politics, Policy and Law* 20 (2): 329–72.

Stevens, Robert, and Rosemary Stevens. 1974. *Welfare Medicine in America: A Case Study of Medicaid*. New York: The Free Press.

Stigler, George. 1988. The Theory of Economic Regulation. In *Chicago Studies in Political Economy*, George Stigler, ed. Chicago: University of Chicago Press.

Stone, Deborah. 1992. Why States Can't Solve the Health Care Crisis. *The American Prospect* 9: 51–60.

———. 1988. *Policy Paradox and Political Reason*. Glenview, IL: Scott, Foresman.

Stonecash, Jeffrey M. 1996. The State Politics Literature: Moving Beyond Covariation Studies and Pursuing Politics. *Polity* 28 (4): 559–79.

Szabo, Joan. 1995. Practice Guidelines: States Lay the Groundwork. *State Health Notes* 16 (No. 195): 4–5.

Taylor, Holly. 1996. Hospitals Find Flaws in Deregulation Proposal. *Albany Times-Union* (April 2): B2.

Thompson, Frank J. 1986. New Federalism and Health Care Policy: States and the Old Questions. *Journal of Health Politics, Policy and Law* 11 (4): 647–71.

———. 1981. *Health Politics and the Bureaucracy*. Cambridge, MA: MIT Press.

Thorpe, Kenneth E. 1993. The American States and Canada: A Comparative

Analysis of Health Care Spending. *Journal of Health Politics, Policy and Law* 18 (2): 477–90.

———. 1989. Health Care. In *The Two New Yorks*, ed. Gerald Benjamin and Charles Brecher. New York: Russell Sage Foundation.

Thorpe, Kenneth E., and Christine Spencer. 1991. How Do Uncompensated Care Pools Affect the Level and Type of Care? Results from New York State. *Journal of Health Politics, Policy and Law* 16 (2): 363–82.

Tierney, John T. 1987. Organized Interests in Health Politics and Policymaking. *Medical Care Review* 44: 89–118.

Tierney, John, William J. Waters, and William H. Rosenberg. 1982. Certificate of Need—No Panacea but Not without Merit. *Journal of Public Health Policy* 3: 178–81.

Traub, James. 1996. Dollface. *The New Yorker* (January 15): 28–35.

Vibbert, Spencer. 1991. New York's Axelrod Leaves Substantial Legacy. *Journal of American Health Policy* 1 (July/August): 58–59.

Vladeck, Bruce. 1981. The Market vs. Regulation: The Case for Regulation. *Milban Memorial Fund Quarterly/Health and Society* 59: 209–223.

Wallack, Stanley S., Kathleen Carley Skwara, and John Cai. 1996. Redefining Rate Regulation in a Competitive Environment. *Journal of Health Politics, Policy and Law* 21 (3): 489–510.

Wallin, Bruce A. 1995. Massachusetts: Downsizing State Government. In Steven Gold, ed. *The Fiscal Crisis of the States*, pp. 252–95. Washington, DC: Georgetown University Press.

Washington Post. 1996. HMOs Issue Guidelines on Patient Information. *Providence Journal-Bulletin* (December 16): A15.

Weiner, Jonathan P., and Gregory de Lissovoy. 1993. Razing a Tower of Babel: A Taxonomy of Managed Care and Health Insurance Plans. *Journal of Health Politics, Policy and Law* 18 (1): 75–104.

Weissman, Joel. 1996. Uncompensated Hospital Care: Will It Be There If We Need It? *JAMA* 276 (10): 823–28.

Weld, William, and Paul Cellucci. 1995. *The Government We Choose: Lean, Focused, Affordable.* Boston: Governor's Office of External Relations.

Wessel, David. 1996. The Outlook. *Wall Street Journal Interactive Edition* (November 11).

Wessner, Connie. 1994a. A Managed Care Experiment: Massachusetts Makes the Grade. *State Health Notes* 15, No. 181 (May 30): 1–2.

Widman, Mindy, and Donald Light. 1988. *Regulating Prospective Payment: An Analysis of the New Jersey Hospital Rate Setting Commission.* Ann Arbor: Health Administration Press.

Wielawski, Irene. 1989. Plan Seems to Split Pie Unfairly. *Providence Journal-Bulletin* (May 27): 1–2.

Wielawski, Irene, Kevin Sullivan, and Katherine Gregg. 1989. Hospital Bailout Plan Blasted by Critics; DiPrete Silent. *Providence Journal-Bulletin* (May 27): 1–2.

Wiggins, Charles, Keith Hamm, and Charles Bell. 1992. Interest Group and Party Influence in the Legislative Process: A Comparative State Analysis. *Journal of Politics* 54 (1): 82–100.

Wilsford, David. 1995. States Facing Interests: Struggles over Health Care Policy in Advanced Industrial Democracies. *Journal of Health Politics, Policy and Law* 20 (3): 571–614.

Wilson, Graham K. 1982. Why Is There No Corporatism in the United States? In Gerhard Lembruch and Phillipe Schmitter, eds., *Patterns of Corporatist Policy Making.* Beverly Hills, CA: Sage.

Wilson, James Q. 1989. *Bureaucracy: What Government Agencies Do and Why They Do It.* New York: Basic Books.

———. 1986. In *Regulatory Policy and the Social Sciences*, Roger Noll, ed. Berkeley, CA: University of California Press.

———. 1980. *The Politics of Regulation.* New York: Basic Books.

———. 1973. *Political Organizations.* New York: Basic Books.

Winslow, Ron. 1992. Strong Medicine: How Local Businesses Got Together to Cut Memphis Health Care Costs. *Wall Street Journal* (February 6): 1.

Winterbottom, Colin, David W. Liska, and Karen M. Obermaier. 1995. *State Level Databook on Health Care Access and Financing*, 2nd ed. Washington, DC: Urban Institute Press.

Winters, Richard F. 1984. New Hampshire. In *The Political Life of the American States*, Alan Rosenthal and Maureen Moakley, eds. New York: Praeger.

Wise, Dan. 1994. HMO Ratings Spur Quality Efforts. *Business and Health* (September): 65–66.

Wong, Doris Sue. 1994. House Democrats Forge a Plan to Delay Health Insurance Mandate. *Boston Globe* (October 14): 37.

Wright, Gerald C., Robert S. Erikson, and John P. McIver. 1985. Measuring State Partisanship and Ideology with Survey Data. *Journal of Politics* 47: 469–89.

York, Myrth. 1997. Making the Deal Go Down Easier. *Providence Journal-Bulletin* (January 1): A7.

Young, David W. 1991. Planning and Controlling Health Capital: Attaining an Appropriate Balance between Regulation and Competition. *Medical Care Review* 48 (3): 261–93.

Young, Oran. 1983. Regime Dynamics: The Rise and Fall of International Regimes. In *International Regimes*, Stephen Krasner, ed. Ithaca, NY: Cornell University Press.

Zimmerman, Harvey, Jay Buechner, and Helen Thornberry. 1977. Prospective Reimbursement in Rhode Island: Additional Perspectives. *Inquiry* 14: 3–15.

Zimmerman, Joseph F. 1981. *The Government and Politics of New York State.* New York: New York University Press.

Zwanziger, Jack. 1995. The Need for an Antitrust Policy for a Health Care Industry in Transition. *Journal of Health Politics, Policy, and Law* 20 (1): 171–73.

Index